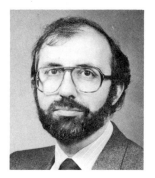

Dr David Chadwick, DM,FRCP is Consultant Neurologist at Walton Hospital, Liverpool, where he runs a large clinic for people with epilepsy. He is also currently involved in an important research project on the effects of drug treatment, which takes him to many other epilepsy centres nationwide. He is married with two children.

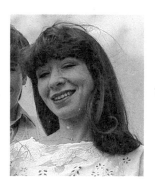

Sue Usiskin was diagnosed as having epilepsy at fifteen. Despite frequent seizures she has adapted successfully to her condition and is married with two children. She is now committed to spreading a truer picture of epilepsy. She talks regularly to groups of medical students about the condition from the patient's viewpoint. She played a large part in the 1980 BBC *Horizon* programme on epilepsy that won the medical programme of the year award.

LIVING WITH EPILEPSY

Dr David Chadwick
and
Sue Usiskin

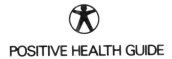

POSITIVE HEALTH GUIDE

I dedicate this book to the memory of my mother, who taught me what courage was all about, and to my dear husband Andrew and children Oliver and Anna for their constant love, support and humour.

SU

© David Chadwick and Sue Usiskin 1987

First published in the United Kingdom in 1987
by Macdonald Optima a division of Macdonald & Co. (Publishers) Ltd.

Revised in 1991

A member of Maxwell Macmillan Pergamon Publishing Corporation plc.

British Library Cataloguing in Publication Data
Chadwick, David *1937-*
    Living with epilepsy.—Rev ed.—(Positive health guide).
    1. Man. Epilepsy. Personal adjustment
    I. Title   II. Usiskin, Sue   III. Series
    362.196853

    ISBN 0-356-19676-3

Macdonald & Co. (Publishers) Ltd
Orbit House
1 New Fetter Lane
London EC4A 1AR

Designed and computer generated in Times by
The Design & Illustration Partnership

Printed in Singapore by
Toppan Printing Company (S) Pte Ltd

CONTENTS

PREFACE

Epilepsy is a common condition that affects millions of people, yet no disorder can claim to be as misunderstood. While heart attacks and even cancer can be discussed openly and frankly today, epilepsy is a subject that is rarely talked about, and one that still carries a considerable social stigma. The reasons for this are understandable. To observers, epileptic seizures can be frightening, confusing, and even violent occurrences, during which people who are outwardly identical to themselves suddenly lose consciousness. They might fall to the floor, possibly injuring themselves and becoming incontinent. The reluctance to discuss the condition perpetuates the misunderstanding, which adds to the burden of epilepsy. This means that people with epilepsy often have to cope not only with their disorder, but also with problems making friends, and making progress at school and at work.

About 1 per cent of the population have epilepsy, so that many people have a friend or relative with the condition. At some time you may witness an epileptic seizure, in the street, in a store or at a big gathering. Everyone should know what this looks like and be able to give the right assistance. Equipped with the proper information, people are less likely to be hostile to epilepsy.

In this book we aim to provide a basic understanding of epilepsy for people with the condition, their families and anyone who has regular contact with them. The information and advice given here will help dispel the myths and misconceptions about epilepsy, and allow people to make commonsense decisions about their everyday lives and activities. We shall show how in spite of epilepsy it is possible to lead an active, enjoyable and relatively unrestricted life.

1 WHAT IS EPILEPSY?

Epilepsy has affected people for as long as history has been recorded. The term is derived from a Greek word that means 'to take hold of, to seize, or to possess'. Although this reflects the ancient Greeks' belief that an epileptic attack represented possession by the gods, by about 400 BC the Hippocratic writers identified epilepsy as a physical disorder of the brain, and pointed out that damage to one side of the brain can lead to convulsions that affect mainly the opposite side of the body. It was defined by the British neurologist Hughlings Jackson a century ago as a recurrent, episodic, uncontrolled discharge of nerve tissue.

How many people suffer from epilepsy?

It is difficult to be certain, but it seems that between one in every two hundred to one in every hundred members of the population – that's 0.5 to 1 per cent – have recurrent seizures at some time in their lives. Fortunately, the majority of these people do not suffer from epilepsy throughout their lives. The illustration on page 10 shows the age-related incidence and prevalence of epilepsy. Incidence is the number of people developing epilepsy for the first time during each year, that is, the number of new cases. Prevalence refers to the number of people suffering from the disorder in any given year; in other words, all new cases plus existing ones. You can see that epilepsy develops most often during the first ten to twenty years of life. Many people developing it at this time do not suffer from seizures during later life. However, some people do go on suffering from the condition for longer periods, and this, taken with the fact that epilepsy develops at a lesser rate in the later years of life, means that prevalence increases with age.

Epileptic seizures and epilepsy

An epileptic attack, or seizure, is a relatively brief episode of altered

9

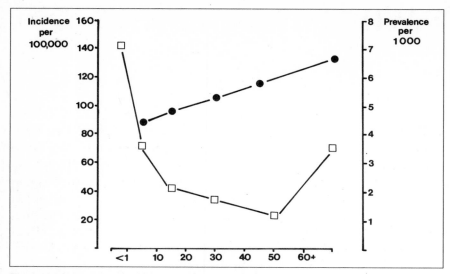

The incidence and prevalence of epilepsy at different ages.

behaviour or consciousness that has a rapid beginning, is usually short and self-limiting, and might be followed by a period of drowsiness and confusion. There are many different types of seizure, and it is important to realize that anyone can have a seizure given the appropriate circumstances. It is the way a normal brain responds to a number of abnormal conditions. For example, someone who develops an infection of the brain – such as meningitis, encephalitis, or a brain abscess – or who has liver or kidney failure, or who takes an excess of any one of a number of drugs, including alcohol, can ha ˙ one or more seizures. Although such a person might have recurr˙ seizures due to his condition, he is not thought of as having epilepsy.

Epilepsy is a disorder of the function of the brain itself, which sometimes results from the scarring of, or other damage to, the brain. So while we all can potentially have seizures, fewer people have epilepsy. To understand the nature of epilepsy, we need to understand the structure and function of the normal brain.

How the brain works

The human brain consists of two cerebral hemispheres with connecting tracts that run through the brain stem into the spinal

10

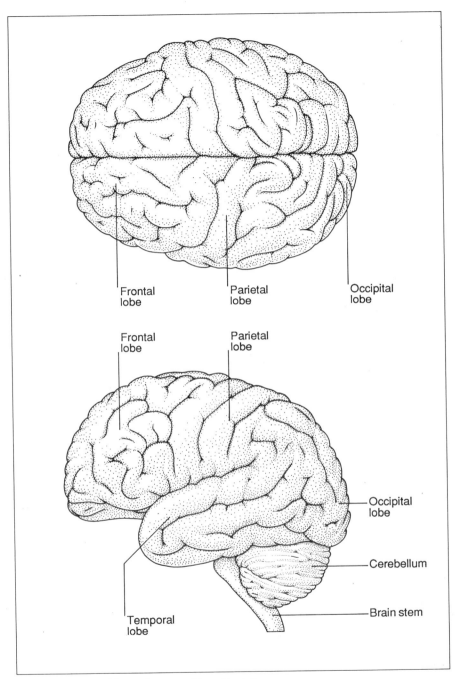

The brain pictured from above and from the left.

cord. The cerebral hemispheres contain large numbers of nerve cells, called neurons, which are responsible for our understanding and perception of the world about us, as well as for the control of our movements and emotions. The nerve cells are interconnected in a vast and infinitely complicated network, and each one can receive messages from hundreds of other cells, and send messages to hundreds more.

Nerve cells communicate with each other by electrical means. When a nerve cell is activated, or fired, an electrical current runs along the nerve fibre and releases a chemical substance, called a neurotransmitter, at the points, or synapses, where it touches other cells. The neurotransmitters can either excite the second cell or inhibit it. If it is sufficiently excited, the second cell will fire, discharging its neurotransmitter to connect with and influence other cells. However, if the second cell receives an inhibitory signal, it will not fire. In this way information is transmitted, integrated and filtered within our nervous system.

A normal nerve cell tends to fire repetitively at a relatively low

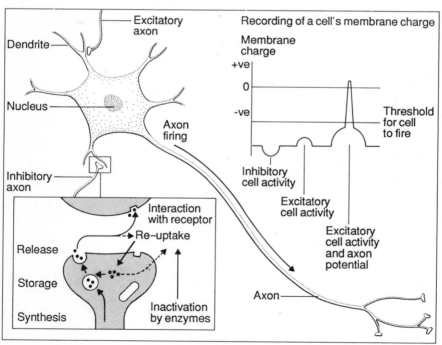

The ways in which nerve cells (neurons) influence each other and their firing.

12

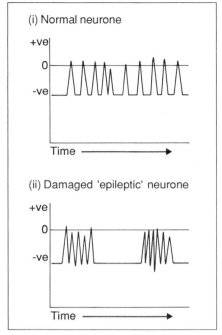

(i) Normal neurone

(ii) Damaged 'epileptic' neurone

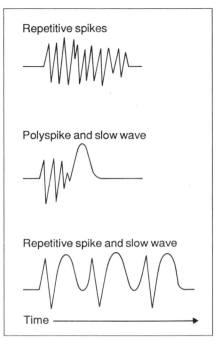

Repetitive spikes

Polyspike and slow wave

Repetitive spike and slow wave

The patterns of activity that can be recorded from (i) a normal cell and (ii) a cell that has been damaged to make it 'epileptic'.

Different types of EEG abnormalities that can be seen in epilepsy.

frequency. If the cell is made epileptic by being damaged, its pattern of firing changes. Instead of discharging at low frequencies, it discharges at extremely high frequencies in bursts. There might be long periods between these bursts when the cell is inactive.

A single cell behaving in this abnormal, epileptic way would not cause anyone to have a seizure. A seizure happens only when many thousands of cells behave in this fashion at the same time. The resulting disturbance may be reflected in the first symptoms of an epileptic seizure, its aura, and may then alter the behaviour of other normal nerve cells, causing the spread of the seizure. When we use an electroencephalogram (EEG) to record changes in the electrical activity, we find that the sudden discharge of several thousand nerve cells usually results in 'spikes', and these are sometimes followed by a slow wave of reduced activity (see above).

Now that we know how an epileptic seizure begins in the brain, we can look at how it affects people.

2 TYPES OF EPILEPTIC SEIZURE

We have seen that a basic abnormality in the function of the nerve cells in the brain leads to a seizure. The brain is so complex that very similar abnormalities in its different areas will produce very different effects in different people. This means that there is an enormous variety of seizures – there probably are as many different kinds of seizure as there are people having them. In spite of this we have to attempt to classify the seizures broadly, because different kinds of seizure can carry very different outlooks (prognoses), have different implications, and require different treatment.

A simplified classification of seizures is shown in the table opposite. The major differentiation is between:

- seizures that begin in a localized part of the brain, which we call partial, or focal, seizures, and

- seizures that affect the whole of both cerebral hemispheres from the beginning, which we call generalized seizures.

We can usually differentiate between these two kinds of fits on the basis of what a person experiences before and afterwards and, perhaps most important, from the description by someone who was there at the time. An EEG can give us further helpful information (see pages 52-5).

Partial seizures

Partial, or focal, seizures begin in a restricted part of one of the cerebral hemispheres. When a seizure discharge begins in this way, the remaining parts of both cerebral hemispheres continue to work normally. The person is conscious but experiences a number of abnormal symptoms, reflecting the normal working of the part of the brain that is affected. This is the warning, or aura, of an epileptic seizure. All attacks of this kind can spread from the site of onset to involve other parts of the brain. In this way both

14

Classification of seizures

Partial seizures (begin locally)

Simple: consciousness not impaired
   a. with motor symptoms
   b. with somatosensory or special sensory symptoms
   c. with autonomic symptoms
   d. with psychic symptoms

Complex: consciousness impaired
   a. beginning as a simple partial seizure and progressing to a complex seizure
   b. impairment of consciousness at onset
      i) impairment of consciousness only
      ii) with automatism

Partial seizures that become generalized (to tonic–clonic seizures)

Generalized seizures

Absence seizures
   a. simple (petit mal)
   b. complex

Myoclonic seizures

Clonic seizures

Tonic seizures

Tonic–clonic seizures

Atonic seizures

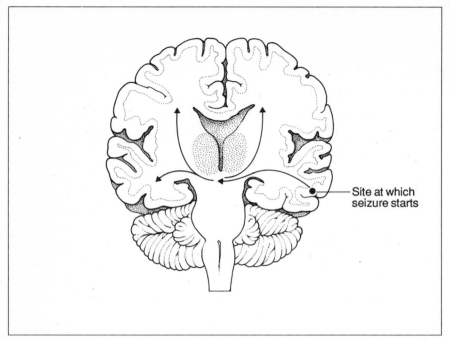

Site at which seizure starts

The onset of a partial seizure in the temporal lobe and the pathways by which it can spread to cause a generalized seizure.

hemispheres can become affected, and a generalized seizure can occur. After a partial seizure is over, symptoms might persist, and they again reflect the part of the brain where the seizure began. The EEGs of people with partial seizures often show that any electrical abnormalities between seizures affect only a particular area of one of the cerebral hemispheres.

What can happen to people during a partial seizure? Let us first consider the partial seizures that are called simple seizures.

Motor seizures

The frontal lobe of each hemisphere controls movement of the opposite side of the body. Therefore, when a seizure begins in the left frontal lobe, movement is produced on the right side of the body, and vice versa. This usually results in what is called an adversive seizure, which affects mainly the head, eyes and arm. In the tonic phase of the seizure (see page 22) the person feels his head and eyes being drawn irresistibly to one side; his hand or arm might become stiff and be drawn upwards. This might be followed by a

16

clonic phase (see page 22), periods of muscular contraction and relaxation that result in the jerking of the head, arm, and leg. Following an adversive fit, people sometimes experience a short-lasting weakness or paralysis, which is known as Todd's Paralysis.

Another type of motor attack is the Jacksonian seizure, named after the British neurologist Hughlings Jackson, who first described it. Although it is rare, it is worth describing here because it shows how seizures can spread from their site of onset. A Jacksonian attack can begin with jerking affecting the thumb of one hand. As the fit spreads, the jerking spreads first to the whole hand, then to the whole arm, then to the face, and finally to the leg. When the jerking involves the whole of one side of the body, the person might lose consciousness and have a typical tonic–clonic seizure (see page 22). If you look at the illustration below, which shows how different parts of the frontal lobe relate to the parts of the body, you can picture how this seizure spreads from its original site of onset.

One of the frontal lobes (usually the left one) is also concerned

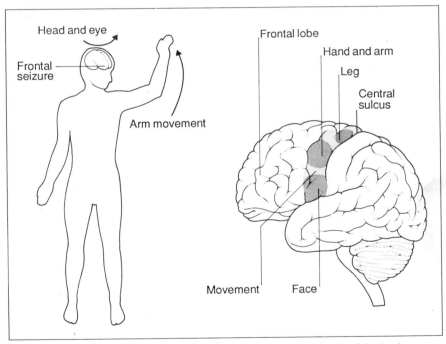

A simple partial seizure arising in the right frontal lobe. The picture of the brain shows which parts of the frontal lobe move which parts of the opposite side of the body.

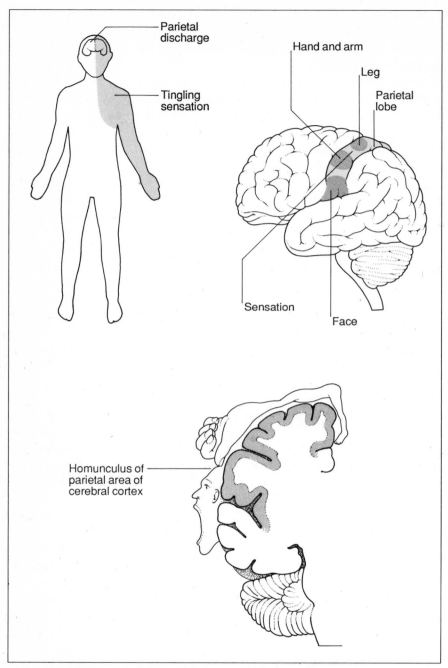

Parietal
discharge

Tingling
sensation

Hand and arm

Leg

Parietal
lobe

Sensation

Face

Homunculus of
parietal area of
cerebral cortex

A simple sensory seizure arising in the right parietal lobe and causing
abnormal sensations on the opposite side of the body.

with producing speech, and sudden 'speech arrest' sometimes occurs during a frontal lobe seizure.

Sensory seizures

The parietal lobe is concerned with physical sensations. When a seizure starts in one of the parietal lobes, a person first feels a tingling, warmth, or other peculiar sensation in a part of the opposite side of the body. Because the part of the parietal lobe that deals with sensation, say in the hand, is intimately connected with the part of the frontal lobe that moves that part of the body, it is quite common for seizures that begin with a sensation also to result in movement. In the same way that motor seizures can be followed by a period of apparent paralysis, sensory seizures can be followed by a period of numbness.

Visual seizures

The occipital lobe at the back of the brain deals with vision. If a seizure begins in this part of the brain, a person experiences abnormal vision, which can be in the form of flashing lights, balls of light, or complicated colours. As in the other types of seizure described above, the experience occurs on the side of the body – in this case, the visual field – opposite to the lobe where the seizure begins.

Simple seizures and the temporal lobe

The temporal lobe is a very common site for the origin of epileptic seizures. Unlike the frontal, parietal and occipital lobes, which have single clearly defined functions in terms of moving, feeling, or seeing, the temporal lobe has many functions. Therefore, when seizures arise in this part of the brain, people can have very varied experiences.

Some parts of the temporal lobe deal with sensations concerned with eating. For this reason seizures that begin here are often associated with a peculiar smell or taste, or an unusual feeling in the stomach. The temporal lobe is concerned with memory too, and some people experience *déjà vu* (the feeling that an event has happened before), or have a recurrent memory that suddenly becomes very vivid; as part of all his seizures one man saw a small boy running along a road picking up pennies. The temporal lobe also deals with our emotions, which is why during such a seizure people might suddenly become frightened, excited or happy.

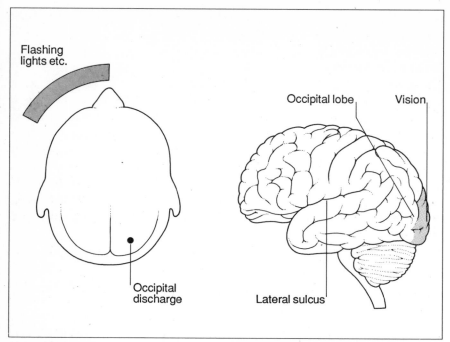

Flashing
lights etc.

Occipital lobe

Vision

Occipital
discharge

Lateral sulcus

A seizure arising in the right occipital lobe. Abnormal visual sensations are
perceived to the person's left.

The distinction between all these simple partial seizures can become
blurred. The division between the different lobes of the brain is
artificial, and some seizures that start in the parietal lobe with a
sensory disturbance will for example spread to the temporal lobe so
that the person may experience a combination of symptoms.

Complex partial seizures

These are the most common kind of partial seizure, and in the past
were called psychomotor or temporal lobe seizures, as they almost
always arise in the temporal lobe. Complex partial seizures differ
from simple partial seizures in that they are associated with some
alteration in consciousness.

Often they begin with the kind of symptoms we have just
described for seizures arising in the temporal lobe. Later, the
person appears to go into a trance during which he is remote,
detached, and out of contact with his surroundings. He may fall, or
appear to go into a sleep-like state for a brief period. Some people
simply appear dazed; others have rather confused behaviour,

perhaps picking at their clothes, smacking their lips, or saying something confused or inappropriate. These actions are called automisms, and a person has no memory of them or of any other event that takes place during his seizure. Occasionally more complicated automisms occur; for example, a person having a seizure in a shop might walk away with an item that he has not paid for. This sort of automism can easily be misunderstood and lead to distressing consequences. All these kinds of complex partial seizure are usually followed by a period during which the person appears confused, not knowing where he is or what he should be doing, before he or she returns completely to normal.

It is thought that complex partial seizures arise because of the spread of abnormal electrical activity from the cortex (or surface) of the temporal lobe into the closely related limbic system. The limbic system consists of a number of structures deep within the temporal lobe and the brain itself that deal with primitive aspects of memory, behaviour and bodily function – so that many temporal lobe partial

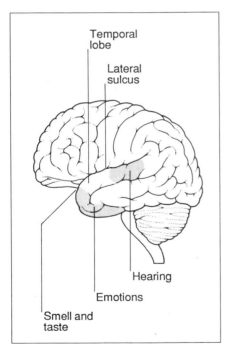

The temporal lobe and some of its functions.

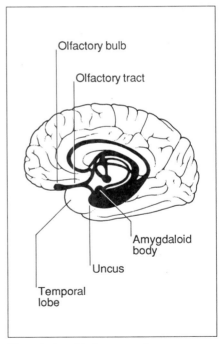

The relationship between the temporal lobe and the limbic system deep inside the brain.

seizures that begin with simple symptoms can become complex during the course of the seizure. Alternatively, if the seizure begins in or very close to the limbic system, the person might lose awareness from the start and not remember any symptoms of a temporal lobe seizure. As we shall see, this kind of seizure can look like petit mal (see page 23). But it is quite different. It is a partial rather than a generalized seizure, and needs different treatment.

Partial seizures that become generalized

One characteristic of the electrical discharge at the basis of seizures is its tendency to spread from the site of onset to other parts of the brain. As we have seen, simple partial seizures can spread to other parts of the hemisphere from where they start. They can also spread to the other hemisphere, resulting in a generalized seizure, which almost always takes the tonic–clonic form. An attack of this kind, that results from spread, is always recognizable because of the particular preliminary symptoms.

Generalized seizures

A generalized seizure is one in which the disturbed electrical activity of the seizure affects the whole of both hemispheres of the brain. It is likely that disturbed activity in the deep structure of the brain is involved in this kind of seizure.

Tonic–clonic (grand mal) seizures

This common type of seizure can arise either because of the spread of seizure activity following a partial seizure, or directly, when it is called a primary generalized seizure. In the former the person suffering the seizure will have symptoms of a partial seizure – an aura – followed by a typical tonic–clonic seizure. In tonic–clonic seizures that are generalized from the start the person does not experience an aura, but loses consciousness immediately.

During the initial tonic phase of the fit all the muscles of the body contract and the person becomes rigid. If his bladder is full, the contraction of the muscles there will result in urination. As the muscles in the lungs contract, they force air out through the vocal cords, and the person seems to cry out. Breathing might stop for a short while, and the person become rather blue as a result. This tonic phase usually lasts for less than a minute, although it might well seem considerably longer, and is followed by the clonic, or jerking, phase. Jerking is caused by phases of relaxation alternating with further muscular contractions. During this part of the fit a person might bite his tongue.

After a minute or two of a clonic phase, the fit ends and the person relaxes. He will then be deeply unconscious and unrousable. Consciousness returns gradually, and within five minutes the individual might be talking, although he will appear rather confused or irritable. He will want simply to be left alone, and might become a little aggressive if interfered with. As consciousness improves, the person will begin to behave more normally, but he might have no memory for forty-five minutes to an hour after the fit. Very often a person remains sleepy and has an unpleasant headache for some time.

There are several other, rarer, types of generalized seizure. They all

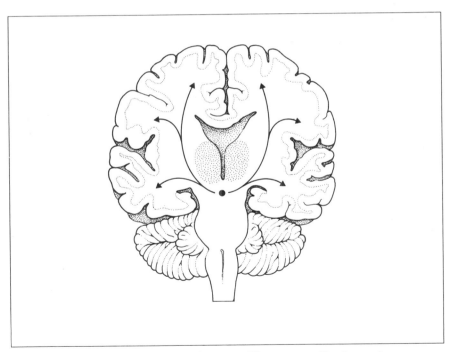

A seizure which is generalized from the onset. The person will not experience an aura.

tend to show themselves first in children, and none of them arises because of spread after a partial fit. Let us consider these in a little more detail.

Simple absence (petit mal)

This type of fit is characterized by a sudden, usually momentary absence during which a child loses contact with his surroundings, stops whatever he or she is doing, and might flutter his or her eyelids. Very often these attacks are so short that they are not recognized by school friends, parents or teachers, and the child who has them is often unaware that they are happening. They can occur many times a day, and sometimes they are so frequent that they interfere with a child's concentration and performance at school.

Everyone is familiar with the term petit mal, but it is often wrongly used to describe any kind of minor epileptic attack. We should avoid this. Simple absences are an unusual and very specific kind of seizure. They should not be confused with other trance-like seizures, such as the more common complex partial seizures, which demand quite different treatment.

Myoclonic jerks

Myoclonus is a sudden, brief, involuntary jerk, which can affect the whole body, but usually involves the arms and sometimes the head. These seizures happen most often in the morning within an hour or so of waking. They are not usually associated with any alteration in consciousness, although sometimes they are accompanied by a brief absence similar to petit mal.

Complex absences

These are seizures that children who often have some underlying brain damage have, and they can recur frequently. The absences are longer than simple absences and much more often associated with either massive jerks or sudden loss of muscle power (atonic attacks), both of which can cause the children to be thrown off their feet. Because of the very sudden onset of the attack and lack of warning, children may injure themselves. Many children suffering this unpleasant kind of attack need to wear protective helmets to avoid head injuries.

When do seizures take place?

Although for a lot of people seizures happen unpredictably, for others patterns of attacks can be identified. Sometimes knowing about these patterns may help precipitating factors to be avoided, so that the frequency of attacks may be reduced.

The sleep–waking cycle
It is not unusual for people to have seizures only while they are asleep. When tonic–clonic seizures happen at this time, they usually have a localized onset; indeed, an EEG recording (see page 52) during sleep is often used to test people who have partial seizures for localized abnormalities.

Some people have generalized seizures, such as myoclonus or tonic–clonic seizures, within an hour or two of waking. They often find that missing sleep is a powerful provocative factor. Attacks tend to take place after a late night, particularly if the person has been drinking alcohol (see page 91).

During the day fits are more likely to occur when people are bored, or apathetic. This should always be borne in mind. Although an active sport such as football might be thought of as slightly risky for a boy with epilepsy, he is more likely to have a seizure if he is sitting indoors by himself while his friends are out playing than if he is out on the football field enjoying himself.

Reproductive cycle
Very often women with epilepsy have seizures related to their menstrual cycle. They usually happen a few days before or just after the beginning of a period. We are not certain why this is. One possibility is that there are changes in the fluid balance of the body and the brain that make seizures more likely during this time. It is also possible that changes in hormonal balance are involved. In spite of this, the oral contraceptive pill seems safe for women with epilepsy and hardly ever has any effect on the occurrence of seizures (see page 83). Taking the drug clobazam in addition to your usual drugs for about five days before and after the first day of a period can sometimes help (see page 64).

Stress factors
Many people with epilepsy say that their seizures are more frequent

When someone is having a fit:

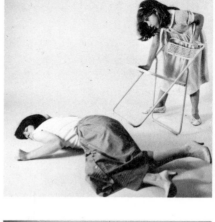

DO

(i) Remove all obstacles near by that could lead to injury.

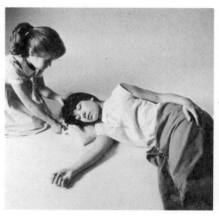

(ii) Turn the person on to his or her side to keep the airways clear and prevent choking. Then place a cushion or any piece of soft material underneath his or her head to prevent unnecessary bruising.

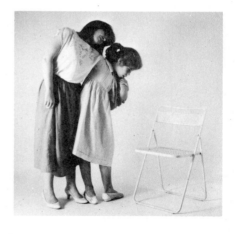

(iii) When the person is ready to get up, lead her gently to a seat and stay with her until she feels all right to move.

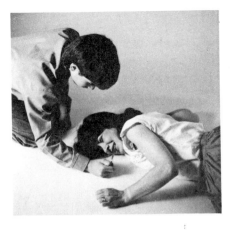

DON'T

(i) Try to force a pencil or spoon between the person's teeth. This will only result in damage to the teeth.

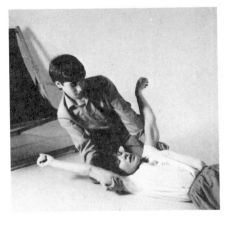

(ii) Drag the person about while the fit is continuing.

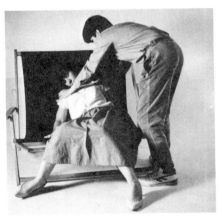

(iii) Force the person to move on to a seat before he or she is ready.

First Aid during and after fits

Do

- Try to move away any objects that might be a danger to the person having the attack. If this is impossible, and only then, you should consider moving the person.

- Try to lay the person down comfortably, usually on the floor or ground, and loosen any tight clothing.

- Try to settle the person comfortably in a semi-prone position on the floor or ground as soon as he is relaxed after the end of a fit. Then leave him to come round slowly. If you interfere with a person during this phase, you might be pushed away or lashed out at in confusion.

- Call an ambulance or a doctor immediately only if someone is having a succession of fits without regaining consciousness between them, which indicates status epilepticus (see page 77).

Don't

- Interfere with a person unnecessarily during a tonic or clonic phase of a seizure. In particular, don't try to introduce spoons or fingers into his mouth in an attempt to prevent him biting his tongue. More damage is usually done by spoons or other implements than by the fit itself.

- Call an ambulance or doctor if someone is having a simple, uncomplicated fit.

and troublesome when they are emotionally distressed or upset. There is certainly an important link between the way people feel and their likelihood of having an attack. Sleep is often disturbed by anxiety or depression, and people may be less consistent about taking their antiepileptic medication when they are depressed.

It must be emphasized that although psychological factors can make seizures more likely if you have epilepsy, they cannot by themselves cause epilepsy, which is a physical disorder.

Reflex seizures

Some people have fits in particular circumstances. Probably the most common of this type of seizure are febrile convulsions. These happen to children up to the age of five only when they have a high temperature (see pages 40-1). Other people are sensitive to flashing lights, which are used as a test to provoke seizures during standard EEG examinations. The usual sources of flashing lights are discotheques and faulty cathode ray tubes in televisions. The flickering television image is particularly powerful in causing seizures. Nevertheless, this kind of trigger is unusual, and working with computers and visual display units (VDUs) is almost always safe.

Now that we have described the common kinds of epileptic seizure, we need to look at the different types of epilepsy – the pattern of recurrent seizures.

3 TYPES OF EPILEPSY

People with epilepsy can suffer more than one type of seizure, and we identify epileptic disorders by the following information:

- the kinds of seizures that occur
- the age at which the seizures started
- whether the epilepsy is likely to be inherited
- the degree to which the cause is identifiable.

It is important to recognize the different patterns of epilepsy because:

- the type of special investigations needed can be different
- the treatment can be different
- the outlook for the control of the condition can vary considerably.

The table opposite is a simplified list of the different types of epilepsy. Let's look first at the generalized epilepsies with seizures that are generalized from the onset. We can subdivide these into:

- idiopathic epilepsies, which are often inherited
- symptomatic epilepsies, which are the result of brain damage or disease.

Idiopathic generalized epilepsies

These are epilepsies with no identifiable cause. People with them have no obvious brain damage or disease and their brains are normal apart from their susceptibility to seizures. It is quite common to find a family history of this form of epilepsy, and it probably has a genetic basis, that is, it can be inherited. These kinds of epilepsy

Classification of the epilepsies

Generalized epilepsies

Idiopathic
   Childhood absence
   Benign myoclonic epilepsy of adolescence
   Tonic–clonic awakening epilepsy

Usually symptomatic
   Infantile spasm syndrome
   Lennox–Gastaut syndrome
   Early myoclonic epilepsies

Partial epilepsies

Idiopathic
   Benign focal motor epilepsy of childhood
   Benign occipital epilepsy of childhood

Sometimes symptomatic
   Simple partial epilepsies
   Complex partial epilepsies

Specific epileptic syndromes

Febrile convulsions

Reflex epilepsies

Stress-induced seizures

Unclassified epilepsies

Neonatal seizures

Nocturnal tonic–clonic seizures (normal EEG)

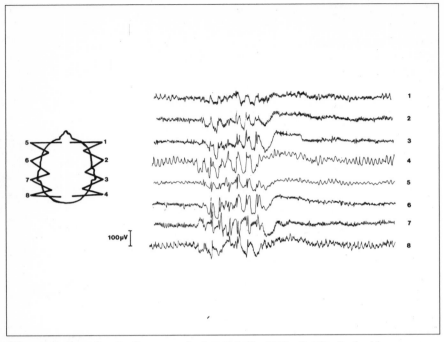

A burst of generalized spike wave discharge in the EEG affecting both sides of the brain simultaneously.

very rarely start before the age of three or after the age of thirty, and the EEGs of people with them show a generalized spike-and-wave disturbance.

Waking tonic–clonic epilepsy

This is the most common idiopathic generalized epilepsy. People have tonic–clonic seizures beginning in childhood or adolescence. There is no specific aura to the attacks, and they tend to be infrequent, and to happen shortly after waking. Treatment for this epilepsy is very effective. It usually ceases soon after medication is started and people may no longer need treatment after fits have been controlled for two to three years. Even if they start again, attacks tend to get less frequent as people get older.

Childhood and juvenile absence (petit mal) epilepsy

This is a much rarer disorder and affects only about 3 per cent of people with epilepsy. Forty per cent of children with this epilepsy have relatives with the condition. They have simple absence

32

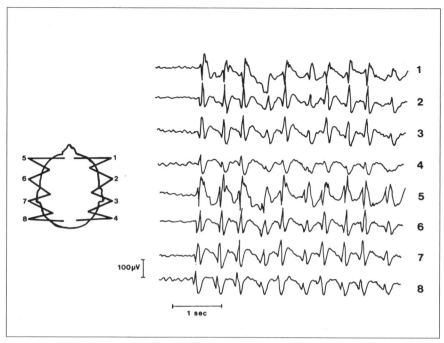

The EEG during a petit mal absence showing synchronous regular spike wave activity at 3 cycles per second on both sides of the brain.

seizures (see page 24), which usually begin between the ages of three and fifteen, and rarely, if ever, continue in adult life, although around one-third of them may have occasional tonic–clonic waking seizures in later life. The disorder shows a very specific EEG abnormality and is characterized by a 3-cycles-per-second spike-and-wave EEG pattern (see the photograph above), and responds well to drug treatment and in the majority of cases people can discontinue therapy in adulthood. Jane's case is a good example.

Jane was seven years old when her parents began to notice that she would stop what she was doing for a second or two, or not reply to a question. They thought that she was daydreaming and were not worried. At first this happened infrequently, but by the time Jane was nine her teachers were concerned about her progress at school, and complained about her poor concentration. One morning while Jane was getting ready for school her mother heard her give a brief cry, followed by the sound of her falling. Her mother ran to the bedroom to find Jane having a convulsion.

The family doctor referred Jane to a paediatric specialist at the local hospital, and an EEG was arranged. It showed that she was having brief absences associated with bursts of 3-cycles-per-second spike-and-wave discharges. There was no doubt that Jane's daydreaming and poor concentration were due to petit mal epilepsy.

Jane was started on treatment with a small dose of sodium valproate. Her parents and teachers were now looking out for Jane's absences, and noticed that they were very greatly reduced. After six months the absences appeared to have stopped. Jane remained very well and a repeat EEG taken when she was twelve was normal. It was decided to withdraw her medication gradually.

Jane's absences did not return and she suffered only two further seizures: a tonic–clonic seizure early one morning when she was nineteen and had been out late at a party the previous evening, and another one when she was twenty-three, six weeks after the birth of her first child.

Benign myoclonic epilepsy of childhood and adolescence

This epilepsy is characterized by early morning myoclonic jerks (see page 24) that affect mainly the arms. Although it is not usually associated with absence, some people do experience brief absence. On some mornings myoclonic jerking might be very frequent and develop into a tonic–clonic fit. The response to treatment is excellent, but prolonged therapy is often necessary, as withdrawal of the drugs can lead to a recurrence of seizures. This is what happened in John's case.

John's father had been discharged from the army because he had had two tonic–clonic seizures at the age of twenty. He had been treated for a brief period with phenobarbitone and had remained well. John was seventeen when he began to experience jerks of his arms soon after getting up in the morning. At first John and his parents assumed this was nothing more than clumsiness, and as he always seemed to improve by the time he had to go to work, they did nothing about it.

John noticed that the jerks seemed to be more of a problem if he had been up late the night before. One Saturday morning after a night out drinking with his friends his jerks were particularly severe, and he decided to go back to bed. Half an hour later his father found John in a confused state, having bitten his tongue and wet the bed.

John's doctor sent him to the hospital for investigation. The neurologist there arranged an EEG. Bursts of generalized spike-and-wave activity showed up and when John was tested by being exposed to a flashing light these became more marked. The neurologist told John and his parents that he had a form of myoclonic epilepsy, and started his treatment with sodium valproate (see page 66). John was told that he would have to give up his provisional driving licence for the present.

To start with, John's morning jerks became far less frequent, but his medication had to be increased before they stopped completely. After two years without a fit John was eager to try to do without his medication, but, unfortunately, soon after reducing the dose he again had morning jerks. John decided to stay on his previous dosage to ensure that he had no further fits and would be eligible for a driving licence.

Symptomatic generalized epilepsies

Children who have suffered some brain damage very early in their lives may have these disorders. They are characterized by many different kinds of seizures, including complex absence seizures, often associated with myoclonus and atonic attacks, and frequent tonic–clonic seizures.

Infantile spasms
This is the most severe and difficult epilepsy occurring in childhood. Attacks usually begin between four and seven months of age, and rarely after twelve months. The most frequent attacks are what are called salaam spasms, when the child's head suddenly and forcefully bends forward while the knees bend and arms flex. Most infants with this epilepsy are brain damaged before they develop these fits, but a few children's retardation is noticed only after the fits have begun. Later the child may have seizures characteristic of the Lennox–Gastaut Syndrome (see below).

The usual antiepileptic drugs have little effect on infantile spasms, but adrenocorticotrophic hormone (ACTH) can be helpful, particularly if treatment is begun early.

The Lennox–Gastaut Syndrome

This begins slightly later than infantile spasms – most often between the ages of one and three years, and rarely after the age of seven or eight. It might account for up to 10 per cent of all epilepsies, and is approximately twice as common as true petit mal.

Children with the Lennox–Gastaut Syndrome have frequent seizures of different kinds. Usually they have complex absence seizures (see page 24), which are often associated with myoclonic jerks, tonic seizures (when the body goes into a spasm), or atonic drop attacks (when the body suddenly loses all its muscular support). They may also have more typical tonic–clonic attacks.

The attacks tend to be much more difficult to control than in true petit mal, and absence status is common. This is a state in which children have a series of absences over a long period, which makes them behave in a confused way. The condition can be very difficult to diagnose unless an EEG is done. There is often mental retardation from an early age, and it can become worse because of the child's

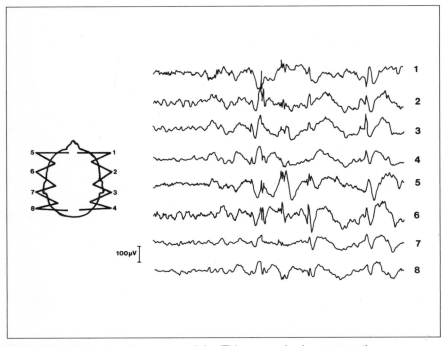

Generalized irregular spike wave activity. This person had symptomatic generalized epilepsy.

epilepsy. Seizures usually continue into adult life, but can sometimes change to become more typical complex partial seizures. Michael's case is typical.

Michael was his mother's first child. She had been in labour for six hours when the midwives became concerned that the baby's heart rate was increasing in an irregular way. Because of this Michael was delivered by forceps, and it was clear that he was far from well. He was taken to the hospital's special baby care unit and placed on a ventilator for four days because he was not breathing very well. During this time he had brief seizures, and was given drugs to suppress them as well as calcium to correct a low level in his blood. Michael gradually improved, and left the hospital two months later.

Michael did not have any further treatment until he was two years old. However, during this time his parents noticed that he was not developing as quickly as they expected. By the time he was two and a half he had not begun to walk, and had been crawling for only three months. His parents became concerned when Michael began to have brief episodes in which he would suddenly jump as though he had been startled, very often falling over. Then he caught a cold and became feverish. His mother found him having a convulsion in his cot and took him to the hospital.

The paediatricians believed Michael had developed a form of epilepsy that was probably caused by brain damage that had occurred around the time of his birth. He was started on drug treatment. Unfortunately although many different drugs were tried, none controlled his fits satisfactorily. He had attacks on most days, and they could occur several times a day. They mostly took the form of brief muscle jerks that would often throw him off his feet. Michael would hurt himself during the attacks, so Michael's doctors arranged for him to wear a special head protector. Less frequently, he had attacks when his body suddenly became stiff and rigid for ten to fifteen seconds. Every two to three weeks he had a tonic–clonic seizure, and after these his parents noticed that his other, more minor seizures were less frequent.

As the years went by Michael's retardation became more obvious, and it was clear that he could not be properly cared for at his local school. He went to a special school, but he never learned to read and write satisfactorily, and he remained very dependent on his parents. By the age of fifteen his attacks had begun to change. He had fewer of the myoclonic attacks and began to have episodes when he would go into a trance-like state and pick at his clothes in an abstracted and fidgety way. His drugs were changed, but while a combination of phenytoin and carbamazepine reduced the number of tonic–clonic seizures he was having to six or seven a year, the new complex partial seizures were still frequent.

A few times Michael became very unsteady and sleepy after an increase in the dose of his phenytoin and the doctors realized he was reacting to the drugs. From then on he had to have regular blood tests to prevent the chances of further drug intoxication.

Michael continued to suffer from severe epilepsy throughout his life. At the age of twenty he was admitted to one of the special centres for epilepsy for a period of assessment and rehabilitation. After this he was able to undertake some light work, which he thoroughly enjoyed.

Partial epilepsies

These make up about 60 per cent of all epilepsies. People with these kinds of epilepsy have partial seizures with or without tonic–clonic attacks. Although they can develop in childhood, they commonly begin at a later age; virtually everyone developing epilepsy after the age of thirty has a partial epilepsy, even those who appear to have only tonic–clonic attacks. Often their grand mal attacks happen when they are asleep and therefore unaware of an aura, which would indicate the localized origin.

Doctors can identify a particular cause for a partial epilepsy more often than they can for a generalized one. It tends to develop after severe head injuries and strokes, and very occasionally is due to a brain abscess or tumour. None the less, in most cases no cause for a partial epilepsy can be found.

Benign focal motor epilepsy of childhood
This is an idiopathic epilepsy in which children between the ages of eight and twelve years begin to have simple motor seizures (see page 16). These are often relatively few and disappear as the child grows up. Tonic–clonic seizures are rare. Some paediatricians

think very mild forms of this kind of epilepsy are so benign that they may not be worth treating. That is what was decided in Mary's case.

Mary woke one night when she was eleven years old because her right hand was jerking. She became frightened when she found she couldn't stop it, and called out to her mother. Almost as soon as her mother arrived in the bedroom the jerking stopped. During the next year a similar sequence of events happened three times, and Mary's parents took her to see their doctor, who sent her to a specialist. Mary's EEG was abnormal with some spikes that were localized over the central region of the left side of the head.

The specialist reassured Mary and her parents that she had a very mild epileptic condition, and emphasized that these kind of attacks continued for a brief period of a person's life and only during sleep. In view of the infrequency of Mary's attacks, he thought that it was not necessary to treat her with antiepileptic drugs. Mary's parents agreed when it was explained that taking drugs might have some minor effects on Mary's concentration and memory. Mary continued to have occasional attacks until she was fourteen, when they stopped.

More rarely, children can have a similar benign epilepsy with seizures arising in the occipital lobe and causing visual disturbance (see page 19).

Children do have other kinds of simple partial epilepsies. These can be caused by brain damage or scarring. They are hardly ever due to serious brain diseases, such as tumours. Although there is a small possibility that a partial epilepsy beginning in adult life could be due to a tumour, the commonest kind – complex partial epilepsy – rarely is.

Complex partial epilepsy
People with this condition suffer from complex partial seizures (see page 20). They might first experience an aura, suggesting an origin in the temporal lobe, followed by a trance-like state and automatism. They might also have tonic–clonic seizures. This kind of epilepsy is important for three reasons.

1. It is very common.

2. Because it is difficult to control completely, it tends to cause more

problems both to people with the condition and their doctors than most other epilepsies. While drug treatment will usually prevent the tonic–clonic seizures, it is often difficult to abolish the trance-like attacks, and about 50 per cent of people with it continue to have attacks and remain on longterm treatment.

3. People who have epilepsy are more likely than other people – and those with complex partial epilepsy are the most likely – to suffer from nervous and psychiatric disorders. Fortunately, these disorders are usually quite mild, but they can include anxiety, depression, and personality problems.

Although there is no simple and certain explanation for the connection between this kind of epilepsy and psychiatric disorders, there are some possibilities:

1. Because complex partial epilepsy is difficult to control, people who have it tend to have more disturbance in their lives, and depression could be a natural reaction to this.

2. Some antiepileptic drugs seem to contribute to psychiatric symptoms, and people with this epilepsy are often placed on larger doses of more drugs than others.

3. As the temporal lobe is important to emotions and other sensations, it is possible that disturbance in this part of the brain is responsible for both an epilepsy and psychiatric problems.

Which are the commonest types of epilepsy? We have already shown how common the condition itself is (see page 9), but it may be interesting to know how many people get which type of seizure. The table opposite shows the results of a study done in Denmark in 1983. Clearly the tonic–clonic seizures make up the largest proportion.

Special situation epilepsies

Febrile convulsions
These happen most commonly to children between the ages of nine and twenty months. The convulsions do not seem to take place before six months or after five years of age. The condition is completely different from other infantile and childhood epilepsies,

Incidence of seizure types

	Per cent
Primary tonic–clonic	25.6
Petit mal	3.9
Myoclonic epilepsies	3.1
Simple partial seizures	4.9
Complex partial seizures	17.9
Partial and tonic–clonic	14.4
Alcohol-induced seizures	6.3
Stress-induced seizures	8.0
Drug-induced seizures	1.3
Isolated unprovoked seizures	13.4
Unclassified	1.2
Total	100

as seizures take place only when children have a temperature higher than 100.4° F (38° C); the normal body temperature is 98.6° F (37° C).

Three per cent of children have febrile convulsions. The susceptibility runs in families, and up to 30 per cent of children suffering febrile convulsions have a near relative who also had them. The attacks usually take the form of tonic clonic seizures, and happen as a fever reaches its peak. Sometimes a convulsion is the first symptom that a child is developing a feverish illness. The convulsions occur usually with simple virus infections, such as coughs and colds, but also with measles and mumps and more serious illnesses, such as pneumonia, gastroenteritis and, occasionally, meningitis. Usually a convulsion takes place only once. Sometimes though there is a repeat, particularly if:

● The first convulsion happened before the age of one year

● The child has had previous brain damage

● Other members of the family have had the same condition.

The chance of children who have febrile convulsions having epilepsy later in life is very low, perhaps as little as 5 per cent. David's case was one of these.

When David was two years old he developed a high fever during a bout of tonsilitis. His mother found him stiff, blue and convulsing. She called the family doctor, who came to the house within twenty minutes. David was still convulsing and the doctor immediately called an ambulance to take him to the local hospital. He was given emergency treatment, which stopped his convulsion, but by that time he probably had been fitting for over an hour. David quickly recovered from this illness and had no further problems until he was ten.

Then David's parents began to notice that he would sometimes stare to one side and swallow. This did not happen often, but when it did, it seemed to upset David. By the time he was fifteen he could describe some of the feelings he experienced at these times: he had a peculiar taste in his mouth, followed quickly by a frightening sensation he couldn't describe. When he was sixteen, his parents found him having a tonic–clonic seizure in his sleep one night.

David was sent to the hospital, where an EEG showed an abnormality in the right temporal lobe. He was told that his attacks were those of a temporal lobe epilepsy, probably caused by damage from his prolonged febrile convulsion. At first he was given phenytoin, and the prescription was later changed to carbamazepine. The drugs reduced the frequency of his attacks to once or twice a month and stopped the tonic–clonic seizures.

David completed his school career successfully, doing well in his examinations, and he went to work for his father as a salesman. But his attacks became longer lasting and more embarrassing. During an attack he would walk about in a confused way, often spitting on the floor. This was followed by quite long periods of confusion, and so it became more and more difficult for him to do his job satisfactorily.

When he was twenty his specialist decided that David should have further, more complex investigations so that the site of onset of his seizures could be discovered. The tests showed that his seizures originated in the right anterior temporal lobe, and it was felt that this could be removed without causing David any harm. After the operation, David had only one more fit, after three months, and years later is taking only a small dose of carbamazepine.

Treatment The first step is to stop the convulsion itself. In most cases febrile convulsions stop of their own accord after a short period. If a child continues to convulse for more than five to ten minutes, you must call a doctor or take the child to the nearest hospital casualty department as quickly as possible. This is important because very rarely febrile convulsions cause brain damage; a high fever seems to increase the possibility of damage to the brain cells during convulsions. The child should probably be taken to the hospital in any case, so that the cause of the fever can be discovered and any possible infection treated.

Should children who have had an episode of febrile convulsions be treated with antiepileptic drugs? Although there is some evidence that taking drugs such as phenobarbitone and sodium valproate may reduce the risk of further convulsions, this seems unnecessary for most children who have had only a single convulsion. All that is needed is for the parents to watch any feverish illness very carefully. You should treat rising temperature by removing the bedclothes and sponging your child with tepid water to keep the body temperature down. Some doctors might also suggest your giving the drug diazepam rectally if a seizure takes place.

Antiepileptic drugs may be necessary for children who are at particularly high risk of further attacks. These are children:

● whose first convulsion happened before the age of one year

● who have shown signs of brain damage

● who have a strong family history of febrile convulsions

● whose first febrile convulsion was particularly long or confined to one side of the body.

Reflex epilepsies
Some people have epileptic attacks brought on by particular circumstances, such as flashing lights. A sensitivity to flashing lights is not common. Only 2 to 3 per cent of people with epilepsy have it, but people suspected of being epileptic are usually exposed to flashing lights in their EEG investigations. Susceptible people show an abnormal EEG pattern. As soon as this appears, the EEG technician can turn off the lights and the person will not realize that

43

anything unusual has happened. However, if a susceptible person is exposed to a flashing light for a longer period, he or she may have a seizure. This is most likely to happen when the person tries to adjust a flickering television set. It can happen when you are driving along a sunlit road with regularly spaced trees, causing dazzling flashes. Although it is extremely rare, pilots who are looking through a nose propeller directly into sunlight can be affected. As we have already said, the flashing lights at a discotheque can also provoke this kind of attack.

Other, much rarer reflex epilepsies are caused by particular sounds or music, or even complicated tasks such as mental arithmetic.

4 DIAGNOSING EPILEPSY

We have seen that there are many types of epileptic seizures, with extremely varied effects, and they can produce unusual and strange sensations. How, then, can your doctor be certain that you have epilepsy? The diagnosis can be very simple and straightforward if you have an aura that is easy to describe, and if your attacks have been witnessed by another person who can describe them to the doctor. An accurate eyewitness account of what happened during an attack is the most useful factor in deciding whether or not you have epilepsy. So it is important for you to try to take an eyewitness with you when you visit the doctor who is investigating any possible epilepsy. You should also be prepared for the doctor's questions, and the checklist on page 46 will be helpful.

Without these clues the diagnosis of epilepsy can be difficult. If you do not have an aura, or have one that is very difficult to describe, and there are no eyewitnesses to your attacks, it might be impossible to reach a firm diagnosis using your account alone. Then investigations may be helpful in coming to a decision. It is best both for you and your doctor to keep an open mind about the nature of your attacks rather than immediately presume they are epileptic. A lot of people have been wrongly diagnosed as having epilepsy: up to 20 per cent of people admitted to special epilepsy centres turn out not to have it, and yet may have had years of inappropriate treatment. The diagnosis of epilepsy has such important implications for the person involved and his or her family that everyone developing symptoms should see a neurologist, paediatrician, or other doctor specializing in epilepsy.

Confusion with non-epileptic attacks

It is important to distinguish between epileptic attacks and other causes of loss or alteration of consciousness.

Checklist: What the doctor wants to know

1. Was there a warning immediately before the attack?

2. Can you describe this warning easily and clearly?

3. Is there an eyewitness who can talk to the doctor?

4. What happened during the attack?

5. How long did the attack last?

6. How did you feel and behave after the attack?

7. Have you had just one kind of attack, or more than one?

8. Have you had any other recent illnesses or symptoms?

9. At the time of the attack had you had any alcohol or taken any drugs?

10. Does anyone else in your family have epilepsy or blackouts?

11. If you have consulted other doctors:
    - who were they?
    - when did you see them?
    - where did you see them?
    - what investigations did you have?
    - what treatment did they advise?

Stroke

Sometimes people are unclear as to the difference between a seizure and a stroke. A stroke is due to a disturbance of blood supply to the brain, and results in an area of brain damage. Its symptoms can come on quickly, but recovery is very slow, usually taking weeks. It is usually older people who have strokes, whereas epileptic seizures are more common among younger ones.

Fainting

Many people have fainted at some time in their lives. It is a normal phenomenon caused by your blood pressure falling to such a low level that it is insufficient to pump blood from your heart up to your head. If your brain does not get enough blood, which carries oxygen, you being to feel lightheaded and quickly become pale, sweaty and slightly nauseated. You may begin to feel that the world is rotating around you, and your vision might become dim, losing the normal appreciation of colour. You will know that you are going to 'black out', and you may feel that you are detached or drifting away.

These feelings are most severe when you are standing up, and are a clear indication that you should lie down. Lying down or putting your head between your knees usually will make you feel better immediately. Too often, however, people feel they need fresh air, and try to walk to an exit, and then they are likely to lose consciousness.

When you faint, you fall to the ground gracefully and rarely injure yourself. Your body is floppy and motionless while you remain unconscious, although some people's bodies jerk once or twice. As soon as you have fallen, your head is on a level with your heart, so circulation to the brain returns and you start to regain consciousness almost immediately. Because of this in the majority of cases there is no confusion between fainting and epilepsy.

Unfortunately, some people are unaware that the act of fainting itself soon restores consciousness, and they will try to help someone who has fainted by picking him or her up. Doing this can prolong the period during which the blood is not reaching the brain, and might even cause the person to have a typical tonic–clonic seizure. This is not an epileptic seizure, and a diagnosis of epilepsy should not be accepted if there is a history of faintness before a seizure.

The differences between fainting and epileptic seizures are listed on page 48. One of the most useful clues is the circumstances in which fainting tends to occur. It is most likely to happen when you are standing still, usually in hot, crowded places such as bars, discotheques, and underground trains. Unpleasant circumstances, such as the sight of blood or an accident, or having an injection can also cause fainting.

Fainting is most common among teenagers and young adults, and is more frequent among women – particularly around the time of their periods – than men. When the cause of fainting is obvious, you do not need to have tests or investigations. However, older people may faint due to dehydration or heart problems, so it is wise to consult a doctor if an old person has fainted. He or she should be investigated and treated appropriately.

Factors differentiating faints and fits

	Faints	Fits
Posture	Upright	Any posture
Pallor and sweating	Invariable	Uncommon
Onset	Gradual	Sudden/Aura
Injury	Rare	Can occur
Convulsive jerks	Rare	Common
Incontinence	Rare	Common
Unconsciousness	Seconds	Minutes
Recovery	Rapid	Often slow
Following confusion	Rare	Common
Frequency	Infrequent	Can be frequent
Precipitating factors	Crowded places Lack of food Unpleasant circumstances	Rare

Hyperventilation attacks

If you have ever had to blow up an airbed without a pump, you will know that taking very deep breaths over a long time can make you feel peculiar. Many people who are anxious tend to overbreathe slightly. When they become particularly panicky, the overbreathing can increase and cause a variety of symptoms that might be wrongly attributed to an epileptic seizure, including:

● Tingling and spasms of the hands

● Nausea

● Lightheadedness and even some alteration of consciousness.

This because overbreathing blows off a gas, carbon dioxide, from the blood. Carbon dioxide concentration in the blood is important in

48

controlling circulation to the brain. Very low concentrations of carbon dioxide cause the blood vessels to constrict and reduce the supply of blood to the head and extremities, producing these symptoms.

Rage outbursts

Although it is true that some people with complex partial seizures experience altered emotions and become confused, violent behaviour during attacks is exceedingly rare. In spite of this, epilepsy is sometimes suggested as the cause when people with short tempers lose control of themselves. Such outbursts of rage are usually provoked, no matter how trivial the cause, and are rarely stereotyped in the way epileptic seizures are. There must be exceptionally firm evidence of an epileptic basis for such outbursts before they are treated as being epileptic.

Pseudoseizures

These are attacks that are feigned, either consciously or subconsciously. They are often used as a means of manipulating people, including the person's family and doctor. For this reason pseudoseizures almost always occur in someone else's presence and they tend to be very dramatic. They are usually less stereotyped than epileptic attacks and often more violent, the arms and legs thrashing about in a very wild manner. They can be particularly difficult to deal with, especially when someone with genuine epilepsy also has pseudoseizures. This is not uncommon and making the distinction between true seizures and pseudoseizures may mean that intensive investigation is necessary.

What are the causes of epilepsy?

Deciding that someone has epileptic seizures is not itself a complete diagnosis because seizures can happen for many reasons. For example, we know that someone who has meningitis may have a seizure. This is not epilepsy; the underlying illness is the cause of the attacks, and successful treatment will also cure the attacks. Chronic epilepsy can be brought on by a number of conditions affecting the brain, some of which are associated with specific age groups. At present we cannot detect a definite cause for epilepsy in about 60 to 70 per cent of cases.

Brain disorders causing seizures and epilepsy

Idiopathic	Inherited epilepsies, other uncertain causes
Congenital	Birth trauma, tuberose sclerosis, arterio-venous malformation
Infections	Meningitis, encephalitis, abscess
Trauma	Severe concussion, haematoma (extradural, subdural, intracerebral), depressed fracture
Tumour	
Stroke	

Neonatal epilepsy
In newborn babies seizures are most likely to develop if:

- There was a problem with the delivery

- The baby has been starved of oxygen

- The baby has low blood sugar or low blood calcium.

Seizures that begin after the first week and during the first year of life often reflect brain damage that occurred before or during birth. Epilepsies in the first year of life starting after the immediate time of birth tend to be relatively severe and difficult to control.

Childhood epilepsies
Epilepsy beginning in a toddler is likely to be a form of generalized epilepsy (see pages 30-8). It can be constitutional and, occasionally, inherited. Infections of the brain are a significant cause for epilepsy at this age, as is brain damage (see Lennox–Gastaut Syndrome, page 36). Epilepsy in a toddler must be distinguished from febrile convulsions (see page 40).

Teenage and adult epilepsies
Idiopathic tonic–clonic and benign myoclonic epilepsies can begin during the teenage years, but not often after the age of twenty-five

or thirty. Then partial epilepsies, which can begin at any age, are the most common type of epilepsy. A person developing partial epilepsy between the ages of twenty-five and sixty may need investigations to exclude the remote possibility of a brain tumour.

Excessive drinking and head injury are common causes of epilepsy at this age, although head injury is an overestimated one. Probably everyone bangs his head at some time, but epilepsy can be attributed to an incident of that sort only if there was a severe injury with prolonged unconsciousness or confusion, or a depressed skull fracture.

Over the age of sixty, the narrowing of the blood vessels appears to be the commonest cause.

Epilepsy and old age
Narrowing of the blood vessels is probably the commonest cause of old people developing epilepsy. Some people develop it as a result of strokes caused by narrowing of blood vessels to the brain. Others have transient ischaemic attacks (TIAs). These are minor strokes that produce short-lasting symptoms, and they need to be distinguished from epileptic seizures.

Distinguishing fits from TIAs is usually very straightforward. TIAs don't generally cause loss of consciousness and they are almost always longer lasting than fits would be. However, if you think an elderly relative is experiencing either fits or TIAs you should ask your doctor. He or she is the person who must differentiate between these two.

People who develop epilepsy in old age have partial seizures, sometimes going on to tonic–clonic seizures. They can usually be treated successfully with drugs, and epilepsy in old age is rarely a major problem.

In the next pages we explain how doctors diagnose the different forms of epilepsy, using special tests.

Testing for epilepsy

If you are suspected of having epilepsy you may need tests or investigations. These will be used to:

1. Help decide whether or not you have epilepsy

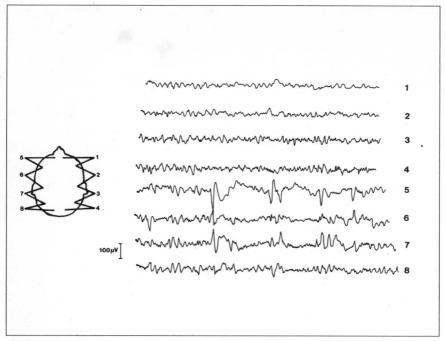

Typical spike discharges arising from the left side of the head. This person had a partial epilepsy.

2. Help decide the kind of epilepsy, which is important in determining treatment.

3. Detect and diagnose a cause of the epilepsy.

EEG investigations

It is unusual for doctors to see someone having a seizure, and equally unusual to be able to make an EEG recording during an attack, which is why a person's medical history and an eyewitness account always form the basis of a diagnosis. An EEG can be useful in adding more weight to a diagnosis of epilepsy, and in classifying it. The EEG by itself is never enough to prove or disprove the diagnosis. Up to 10 per cent of people who have never had an epileptic fit have mildly abnormal electrical patterns, and some people who have epilepsy have normal EEGs between their attacks. Still, since many people with epilepsy show abnormal EEG patterns between their attacks, this is a useful test.

An EEG is a very simple and painless procedure that should not

52

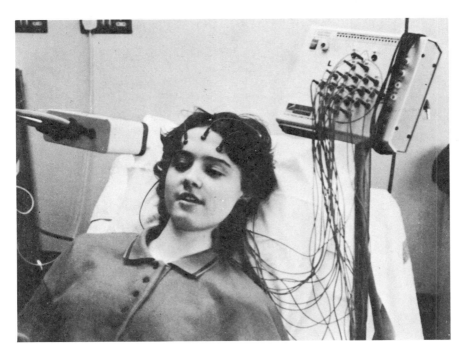

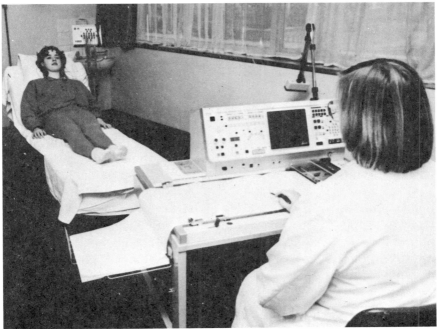

Recording the EEG.

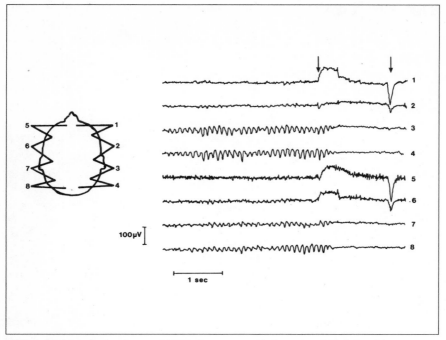

A normal EEG pattern. The regular activity in channel 3, 4, 7 and 8 is a normal alpha rhythm that occurs when someone lies still with closed eyes. The large waves marked by the arrows indicate eye movements, the first of which is associated with opening of the eyes which abolishes the preceding alpha rhythm.

cause you any stress or worry. We have seen that the brain works through networks of nerve cells that communicate with each other by electrical signals (see page 12). The EEG detects and records this activity on paper; it should not be confused with electroconvulsive therapy, when electricity is administered to the brain as a treatment for depression.

When you have an EEG, you will have up to twenty metal tags lightly glued to your scalp. This allows up to sixteen simultaneous recordings, or channels, from different parts of the brain. Sometimes the person's scalp is gently scratched beneath the tags to improve the recording. Because the electrical activity of the brain is difficult to detect and is easily obscured by any movement or muscle activity around the scalp, you will be asked to lie very still on a couch in a quiet environment. The recording takes about twenty to thirty minutes. At some point you might be asked to open and close your eyes, and to breathe deeply and regularly for a period of up to three minutes. The technician might flash a strong light in your eyes. This is done to see if abnormal patterns are produced that would not otherwise be detected. If an abnormal pattern does develop, the technician will stop this part of the test to make sure that a seizure is not provoked. Sometimes EEGs are recorded during sleep, as particular kinds of epileptic abnormalities are more likely to occur then.

A normal EEG pattern is shown opposite. You can compare it with the abnormalities in the records from a person with a partial epilepsy (see page 38), and you can compare both of them with abnormal records from people with generalized epilepsies (see pages 30-8).

For most people with epilepsy, a standard EEG is the only test necessary. However, recording the brain waves for twenty to thirty minutes is unlikely to result in an attack being recorded. If there is doubt about the nature of someone's attacks, more prolonged testing is necessary so that an actual attack can be recorded. Two new systems for longer recording of EEGs now make this possible.

Telemetry   For this you remain in a room under constant observation by a video camera. At the same time an EEG is recorded on magnetic tape. These recordings can be continued for days at a

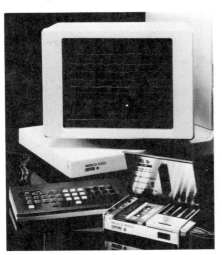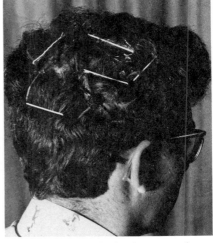

Ambulatory monitoring equipment. *Left,* the cassette recorder in the foreground has a tape in place ready for recording. The monitor in the background shows the display from a tape which has been previously recorded. *Right,* the leads are in place, with hair clipped back to demonstrate. The hairgrips would be removed and the hair smoothed down so that they would usually be invisible during recording.

time, so it is possible to compare the videotape of your activity with the pattern of EEG during an attack.

Ambulatory monitoring Telemetry is done in an artificial situation and so the results may still be ambiguous. A new system of ambulatory monitoring allows testing in more natural circumstances. It records six to eight EEG channels, instead of the usual sixteen, on a portable tape recorder similar to a Walkman. After you have been into the recording unit to have the electrodes attached and the tape recorder turned on, you can leave the hospital and continue your normal routine. The tape can later be read with special equipment back at the hospital.

X-ray and imaging tests
The vast majority of people with epilepsy need few investigations other than an EEG. Sometimes, however, x-ray investigations are necessary to help determine whether scarring of, or an abnormality in, the brain is responsible for the epilepsy. Ordinary x-rays of the

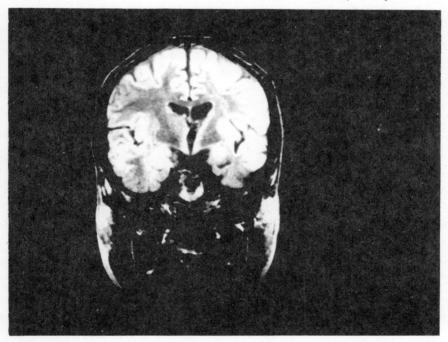

A magnetic resonance scan showing the left half of the brain responsible for a patient's complex partial epilepsy.

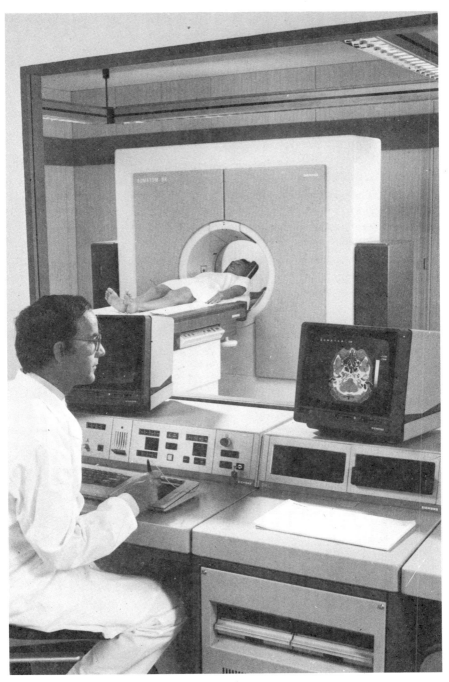

CT scanning

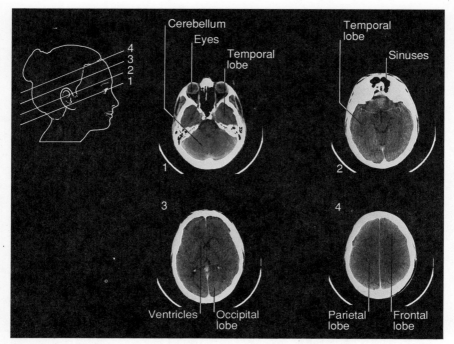

A normal CT scan showing the brain can be visualized by this test.

head do not help because they show only the bones of the skull. To obtain information about the structure of the brain some form of brain scanning is needed.

The most widely available kind of brain scan is the isotope scan. In this test a mildly radioactive isotope is injected into a blood vessel in your arm. As the blood circulates, it carries the isotope to the brain. A special gamma camera, which is sensitive to the small amount of radiation emitted by the isotope, is used to photograph the isotope's passage through the brain. The isotope shows up as a dark image on the photograph, or scan; the darker the image, the greater the amount of isotope present. This technique helps detect areas of the brain with a particularly active blood supply, as well as abnormal blood vessels and some kinds of tumours that can cause epilepsy. However, it cannot detect many other kinds of scars that can cause seizures.

The type of scanning that gives us the most information is called computerized tomographic (CT) scanning. You simply lie on a table and your head is placed in a specialized x-ray machine. The machine takes two-dimensional x-ray pictures of your head from a

58

great many angles. The results are processed by a computer to produce an image of your brain, which shows tremendous detail. A scan of a normal brain is shown opposite. CT scanning can show up a variety of cysts, scars, and abnormal blood vessels in the brain, and can help identify the rare cases when people have some kind of tumour causing their epilepsy.

A new kind of scanning that will become very important for people with epilepsy is magnetic resonance imaging (MRI). This is a revolutionary new technique in which a person lies with his or her head within a large, very powerful circular magnet. Images are produced by changes in the magnetic field which are analysed by a computer used to construct images of the brain. No x-rays are involved in this technique and it produces very high quality pictures. This form of scanning is not yet widely available for people with epilepsy but it already seems that it may be better at showing up areas of scarring in the brain than is CT scanning. It will be some time before we fully understand how important this test may be for people with epilepsy.

Blood tests are less helpful. They can be used to detect low blood sugar, low blood calcium, and evidence of infection and kidney or liver failure, but they are not necessary for most people. Anyone whose epilepsy is caused by one of these problems will probably have many complaints other than just seizures and so will have to have a series of thorough tests.

Is retesting ever necessary? Once initial tests have been completed, it is not often necessary to have repeat tests. Occasionally further EEGs are helpful, if:

● treatment is not being as effective as expected

● new symptoms develop

● stopping drug treatment is being considered.

In the next chapter we describe the different types of treatment available, and which you are most likely to be given according to the sort of seizures you have. We also talk about the chances of doing without drugs after a period of treatment - when and for whom this is possible.

5 TREATING EPILEPSY

Epileptic fits can be dramatic and frightening events. People seeing one for the first time feel an understandable desire to interfere and to try to protect the person having the attack. It is important to remember that seizures are self-limiting and that, in the vast majority of cases, people are not seriously injured. The list on page 28 explains what you should and should not do to help someone having a seizure.

Most people who have epilepsy need to take drugs to prevent further attacks. The success of your treatment depends on your taking medication regularly; forgetting to do this is perhaps the commonest reason for treatment failing. Many people do not have any further attacks after they start the treatment.

When to start antiepileptic drugs

In the past people were sometimes given antiepileptic drugs even before they had a seizure. People who suffer very severe head injuries or who have particular kinds of neurosurgical operations do have a high risk of developing epilepsy, and so at one time neurosurgeons gave them antiepileptic drugs. However, there is little evidence that starting treatment at this stage prevented the development of epilepsy, and it meant that many people were receiving unnecessary medication.

We know that having one seizure does not mean that someone has epilepsy. As many as 70 per cent of people who have not had a second attack within six to eight weeks of their first will never have another. For this reason it is now usual not to treat people until they have had at least two epileptic seizures. Even some people who have had two seizures will not need treatment. Each case needs very careful consideration. Most doctors probably would not start treatment if a person's attacks were very infrequent, perhaps less than one every one to two years. Some people who have had more frequent attacks might not need treatment if a clear provoking factor

Starting antiepileptic treatment

Problem	Usual clinical practice	Modifying factors
Prospective risk of epilepsy	No treatment	
Single isolated seizure	No treatment	Progressive cerebral disorder. Clearly abnormal EEG.
Two or more seizures	Monotherapy	Seizures more than 1 year apart Identified precipitating factors (drugs, alcohol, photic stimuli) Patient acceptance

can be identified. For example, children with febrile convulsions (see page 40), or people who have fits provoked only by flashing lights or by alcohol withdrawal usually do not need treatment; they and their families simply need advice about avoiding the provoking factors.

A person's attitude towards treatment is also important, and if you feel any reluctance about accepting it you should discuss this frankly with your doctor.

Choosing the right drug

The aim is always to control epilepsy with the simplest possible drug regime that has the fewest side effects. Therefore it is usual to begin treatment with a small dose of a single drug. In many cases this stops attacks; the dose will be increased gradually only if you have further attacks. Your doctor will decide which drug to give you after very careful consideration of the following:

1. Which drugs are likely to be most effective against the kind of epilepsy you have?

2. Which of the effective drugs is likely to have the fewest side effects?

3. Which of the effective drugs will be easiest for you to take?

61

The drugs used to treat epilepsy, the kinds of epilepsy for which they are used, and their more common side effects are summarized in the table on pages 64-6.

Payment for drugs and further assistance
In the UK people with epilepsy are exempt from prescription charges for antiepileptic drugs. You should get leaflet P11 from the Post Office, and fill in Form C and send it to your doctor to sign. If your fits are so frequent that you need attendance during the day and night, you might be able to obtain an attendance allowance. Information and instructions on how to claim can be obtained from your Social Security Office.

There are a number of epilepsy associations, which provide information, advice, and social contacts for people with epilepsy, and raise money for research. They are listed on page 119.

Names of drugs
Many drugs have at least two names. The chemical, or generic, name is given first in the table and the text, and the proprietary, or trade, name is given second. For example, phenytoin is the generic name of the drug that is sold as Epanutin by the manufacturer Parke-Davis. A pharmacist might provide either the generic or the proprietary drug when a prescription is made out for the generic, so you might be given either phenytoin or Epanutin if your doctor has prescribed phenytoin. In the case of phenytoin it is important that people are not changed from the generic to the proprietary drug or vice versa, as differing amounts of the drug pass into the body from the two formulations. The differences between generic and proprietary versions of other drugs are not so crucial.

Indications
This tells you for which kinds of epilepsy a drug is used. The table describes usage in three ways.

1. Drug of choice: also called a 'first line' drug; that is, the preferred one

2. Effective drug: a 'second line' drug, used when the drug of choice is not available or not satisfactory

3. Occasional use: a drug that might be used, but usually only when the first and second line drugs have proved unsatisfactory.

Side effects

Many drugs produce side effects, and these are categorized in the table as follows:

- Dose related: effects that anyone can have, given high enough doses, but which will disappear when the dose is reduced

- Allergic: reactions that occur rarely, unpredictably, and usually soon after the drug is started, and will recur if it is taken again; many reactions such as rashes are true allergies, but the ways that others develop are less certain

- Chronic toxicity: effects that develop slowly, after prolonged use; these are more common in people taking large doses of more than one drug.

The commonest dose-related side effect is intoxication, or 'drunkenness'. Particularly with phenobarbitone, phenytoin, primidone and carbamazepine, this can cause sleepiness, difficulty with concentration, unsteadiness in walking, and slurred speech.

Older drugs tend to have more side effects than the more recent ones. For example, many people who take phenobarbitone and to a lesser degree phenytoin, even in moderate doses, feel rather tired, sleepy and sedated, and we can measure the adverse effect on memory, alertness and reaction time. The newer drugs carbamazepine and valproate have fewer effects of this nature and so are usually preferred. Phenobarbitone, primidone and phenytoin can have unpleasant cosmetic effects, causing acne and facial hairiness, which is unpleasant for women. Phenytoin can also be difficult to use because even quite small increases in the dose can cause a large rise in its concentration in the blood, and symptoms of intoxication. Frequent blood tests are usually necessary to check the concentration of phenytoin, whereas this is not necessary with carbamazepine and valproate.

What should you do if you have side effects?

If you develop 'drunkenness' you should go and see your own doctor, who will advise you about changing the drug dosage. It's not necessary to change the drug itself. These symptoms should settle within a few days of the change in your dose.

If you forget a dose of your drug, with drugs such as phenytoin, phenobarbitone and valproate you can take the next two

Generic name	Trade name	Maker	Indications	Adverse effects	Dosage	Optimal serum concentration	Interactions	Preparation
Carbamazepine	Tegretol	Geigy	Drug of choice: complex partial seizures, particularly if complicated by psychiatric disturbance, tonic–clonic and simple partial seizures	Dose related: dizziness, double vision, unsteadiness, nausea and vomiting Allergic: rashes, reduced numbers of white blood cells Chronic toxicity: few known - absence of major effects on intellectual function and behaviour is major benefit	300–1600 mg/day – can be given in 2 or 3 doses. Initial dosage should be low, with slow increments. Early intolerance is common if dose is increased too quickly.	4-10 µg/ml, but little evidence to substantiate this. Blood level monitoring not essential.	Increases rates of breakdown of oral contraceptives, phenytoin, valproate, all of which may need to be given in higher doses with tegretol. Levels of carbamazepine usually lower when given with other drugs.	100, 200, 400 mg tablets, 100 mg/5 ml syrup
Clobazam	Frisium	Hoechst	Occasional use: tonic–clonic and partial seizures particularly if occurring at period times in women. (Value is greatly limited by development of tolerance)	Dose related: drowsiness and sedation	Up to 30 mg/day in 2 or 3 doses	Uncertain		10 mg tablets
Clonazepam	Rivotril	Roche	Drug of choice: status epilepticus Effective in: absence, myoclonus Occasional use: tonic clonic and partial seizures (Value is greatly limited by development of tolerance; that is, its effects wear off as a patient becomes used to the drug)	Dose related: sedation, inflammation of veins if given intravenously	Orally 0.5–4 mg 3 times a day, in slowly increasing doses	No obvious correlation with therapeutic effect. Not routinely measured.	Combination with valproate may exacerbate absence seizures.	0.5, 2.0 mg tablets, 1 mg ampoules for intravenous injection.

Generic name	Trade name	Maker	Indications	Adverse effects	Dosage	Optimal serum concentration	Interactions	Preparation
Diazepam	Valium, Diazemuls, Stesolid	Roche, Kabi-Vitum, CP Pharma-ceuticals	Drug of choice: status epilepticus Occasional use: absence, myclonus (Value is greatly limited by development of tolerance)	Dose related: sedation	Intravenous. Rectal administration may be of value when intravenous is not practical. Not very effective taken orally.	Uncertain		Valium 2 mg, 5 mg, 10 mg tablets, 2 mg/5 ml syrup, 10 mg ampoules for I/V injection Diazemuls 10 mg ampoules for I/V or rectal administration Stesolid 10 mg tubes for rectal administration
Ethosuximide	Zarontin, Emeside	Parke-Davis, Laboratories for Applied Biology	Drug of choice: simple absence (petit mal)	Dose related: nausea, drowsiness, dizziness, unsteadiness, may exacerbate tonic–clonic seizures Allergic: rashes	Up to 2 g/day in 2 or 3 doses	40–100 µg/ml		250 mg capsules, 250 mg/5 ml syrup
Phenobarbitone	Gardenal, Luminal, Prominal	May and Baker, Winthrop, SK and F	Effective in: tonic–clonic and partial seizures Occasional use: status epilepticus, absence	Dose related: drowsiness, unsteadiness Allergic: rashes Chronic toxicity: tolerance, habituation, withdrawal seizures. Adverse effects on intellectual function.	Up to 200 mg/day orally, in 2 or 3 doses	15–35 µg/ml but upper and lower limits modified by development of tolerance.	Combination with valproate may cause drowsiness. In combination it may lower levels of phenytoin and carbamazepine, and oestrogens from the oral contraceptive.	15 mg, 30 mg, 60 mg, 100 mg, 200 mg tablets, 30 mg/10 ml elixir, 60 mg, 100 mg spansules
Phenytoin	Epanutin	Parke-Davis	Drug of choice: tonic–clonic, simple and complex partial seizures	Dose related: drowsiness, unsteadiness, slurred speech, occasionally abnormal movement disorders Allergic: rashes, swelling of lymph glands, hepatitis Chronic toxicity: gum swelling, acne, coarsening of facial features, hirsuitism, folate deficiency	200–600 mg/day in 1 or 2 doses	10–20 µg/ml. The relationship between dose and serum concentration necessitates frequent blood level monitoring.	Its metabolism is inhibited by sulthiame, and its protein-binding by valproate. Tends to reduce blood concentrations of other antiepileptic drugs and oral contraceptives.	25 mg, 50 mg, 100 mg capsules, 50 mg chewable tablets, 30 mg/5ml suspension

Generic name	Trade name	Maker	Indications	Adverse effects	Dosage	Optimal serum concentration	Interactions	Preparation
Primidone	Mysoline	ICI	Occasional use: tonic–clonic and partial seizures	Dose related: drowsiness, unsteadiness. Often tolerated poorly on initiation and a slow increase in dose is advisable. Allergic: see phenobarbitone Chronic toxicity: see phenobarbitone	500–1500 mg/day in 2 or 3 doses	As phenobarbitone; it is changed in the body to phenobarbitone.	See phenobarbitone. Phenytoin and carbamazepine increase the transformation to phenobarbitone in the body, and may precipitate intoxication.	250 mg tablets 250 mg/ml suspension
Sulthiame*	Ospolot	Bayer	Occasional use: tonic–clonic and partial seizures	Allergic: breathlessness, weight loss Chronic toxicity: pins and needles in hands and feet	200–800 mg/day in 2 or 3 doses	Uncertain	Prevents breakdown of phenytoin and causes a rise concentration in blood. Is probably only weakly antiepileptic when given alone or with drugs other than phenytoin. This and toxicity limit its use.	50 mg, 200 mg tablets 50 mg/5ml suspension
Troxidone	Tridione	Abbott	Effective in: absence seizures	Dose related: diplopia, drowsiness, vertigo Allergic: rashes, photophobia, bone marrow suppression, kidney damage, hepatitis. Toxicity means that this drug is very rarely used	300–1800 mg/day in 2 or 3 doses	Uncertain		300 mg capsules
Valproate	Epilim	Labaz	Drug of choice: all idiopathic generalized epilepsies Effective in: partial and secondary generalized epilepsies	Dose related: tremor, irritability, restlessness, occasionally confusion Allergic: gastric intolerance, liver damage Chronic toxicity: weight gain, hair loss	600–3000 mg/day in 2 or 3 doses	Uncertain: blood levels vary a lot during the day and a single specimen is unreliable.	Serum concentrations fall with phenytoin and carbamazepine. May increase phenobarbitone levels when given in combination with phenobarbitone or primidone.	100 mg (crushable), 200 mg, 500 mg tablets 200 mg/5 ml syrup and elixir
Vigabatrin	Sabril	Merril Dow	Effective in partial epilepsy	Dose related, may cause confusion and psychosis occasionally	1000–3000 mg/day in 2 doses	Not relevant.	Can cause a fall in phenytoin concentrations.	500 mg tablets

* This drug has been withdrawn from the market but may still be available if the doctor prescribing it feels that the person cannot be controlled by anything else (this is called a named patient prescription).

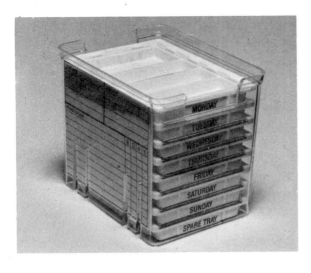

A medication organizer can help you remember to take your tablets. Discuss the idea with your doctor before starting this system.

doses together. With a drug like carbamazepine, taking two doses together may cause side effects and with this drug I usually tell people who have forgotten not to worry and just to take the next one when they should.

You certainly must tell your doctor if you are missing medication regularly. You may find it helpful to get one of the little boxes that can be divided up so that you can put the week's supply in. Then you can be sure you actually take your pills on the day and at the time when you should.

Optimal serum concentration
It is now possible to measure the concentration of a drug in a sample of blood. For many drugs we can define a range of levels below which there might be room for increased dosage and improved control of seizures – but above which there is an increased risk of side effects. Having this measurement taken can ensure that you are being given the correct dosage.

Treatment for continuing seizures

A few people will continue to have seizures after they have started taking antiepileptic drugs. They are most likely to be people who have partial seizures, particularly those with complex partial epilepsy. What can be done in this situation? It is certainly

67

reasonable to increase the dose of the original medication cautiously until either the attacks disappear or side effects begin to develop. By having blood tests regularly to check the concentration of the drug, it is often possible to predict when side effects might develop (see page 63).

With increased doses of drugs tonic clonic seizures usually become less frequent and might stop, but sometimes it is difficult to prevent partial seizures taking place. Then the possibility of changing to another drug or of adding a second drug and having a trial period when you take a combination of drugs will have to be considered. However, it is unusual for either of these alternatives to improve control dramatically where a single drug has failed.

Doctors try to avoid combining drugs. Taking two, three or even four different ones can cause many problems. They can interact with each other, and you are certainly much more likely to have side effects if you take a combination. Each drug can also interfere with the action of the others, so that it can be difficult to obtain satisfactory concentrations of drugs in the blood. Since there is no good evidence that people are better off on two drugs rather than one, let alone three rather than two, there is a powerful argument for keeping treatment simple and restricting it to a single drug whenever possible.

It is important to understand what expectations we can realistically have of drug treatment. Sometimes it can be extremely difficult to abolish a person's attacks completely and if your doctor has explained that this is true in your case, it would seem sensible to accept the best compromise by which you have some attacks but avoid too many side effects from your medication. The need to limit treatment to a level that can prevent, for example, major tonic–clonic seizures and restrict the number of more minor seizures to an acceptable level, while avoiding your having to walk around in a zombie-like state, needs to be discussed and fully understood both by you and your doctor.

Should you stop treatment?

Doctors treating epilepsy have very clear ideas about beginning and continuing therapy, but, perhaps, less often consider stopping treatment or limiting the amount of medication used. These possibilities are very important to people with epilepsy. As many as

70 to 80 per cent of people with epilepsy will stop having seizures very soon after they begin treatment. Should they continue to take drugs for the rest of their lives, thereby running the risk of side effects, or should they be advised to stop their treatment?

It is usual to continue treatment for at least two to three years before considering this. Even then the question is very difficult to answer. We know that approximately 20 per cent of people who develop epilepsy during childhood, and approximately 40 per cent of those who develop it during adult life, will have further seizures if medication is stopped after a two-to-three year period free of attacks. At present doctors do not have enough information to predict accurately who can safely stop treatment, and who needs to continue it. The people who are likely to be at greatest risk of suffering further seizures if they stop taking drugs are those:

● Who develop epilepsy in later life

● Whose epilepsy is related to an identified cause

● Whose epilepsy has been difficult to control in the past.

Before any decision is made to withdraw drugs, you and your doctor should discuss all the risks and possible benefits of this action. Perhaps the most important factor in reaching a decision is your own attitude. Some people feel very insecure at the thought of stopping their treatment; others that taking medication is inherently bad, and are happier without treatment if at all possible. On the one hand, drivers have to take the risks of further seizures most seriously; in the UK a single seizure after stopping treatment will result in the loss of your driving licence for at least two years. On the other hand, women should consider a trial of drug withdrawal before pregnancy so as to have the best chance of a pregnancy free from drugs and seizures. Each person has to make his or her own appraisal and decision.

If you are stopping medication this should be done slowly and gradually; stopping suddenly can produce withdrawal seizures. There are no hard and fast rules about how you do it, but perhaps reducing the medication by a tablet per day at two to four weekly intervals, with the aim of stopping treatment no sooner than three to six months after you begin the reduction, would be a reasonable approach. In any case, this should be done with your doctor's advice.

Stopping antiepileptic drugs

Absolute requirement	Factors in favour	Factors against
Minimum of 2 years fit-free	Childhood epilepsy	Late onset epilepsy
Patient's informed consent	Primary generalized epilepsy	Partial epilepsy
	Idiopathic epilepsy	Symptomatic epilepsy
	Short duration	Long duration
	Normal EEG	Abnormal EEG
	Non-driver	Driver

If you stop your tablets too suddenly and without medical advice you may get withdrawal seizures. Provided you really want to persevere off treatment, it might be worth carrying on – but again, you must talk to your doctor about it. In most circumstances further seizures on withdrawal mean going back on treatment is necessary.

Other kinds of treatment

As we have seen, the fact that someone has epilepsy is not a diagnosis in itself as the condition can have many causes. For this reason people who develop seizures may need other treatments in addition to their antiepileptic drugs. These range from counselling and psychiatric treatment for people who have been drinking alcohol excessively, or taking antibiotics to control infection for people with meningitis or an abscess, to operations for cysts and tumours.

An operation to control epilepsy is possible for some people for whom drugs have proved unsuccessful. Two different kinds of approaches are used. Most commonly an operation aims to remove that part of the brain where the seizures begin. Such operations usually remove part of the temporal lobe but some operations can be made on other parts of the brain as long as there is no risk to the individual person's physical and mental well-being. A second type of operation does not remove any of the brain but divides the connections between various parts of the brain (callosotomy or multiple subpial resection). This second kind of operation is much more rarely done.

There are relatively few operations performed for epilepsy in the United Kingdom but this kind of treatment is becoming more widely available in some specialist centres in the United Kingdom, and is much more commonly used in the United States. As many as 50–70 per cent of people who have operations for epilepsy can be cured whilst perhaps another 10–25 per cent are very much improved. The results of the operation are never, however, 100 per cent guaranteed and every individual person needs to be considered very carefully before a decision to operate is taken. Many specialized EEG tests need to be undertaken which have to include recording of the seizures so as to pinpoint where they start and how they spread. Specialized tests of memory and speech will usually be needed to make sure that these functions will not be harmed by an operation.

Other kinds of treatment are used even more rarely. A ketogenic diet, which is rich in fats and oils, is sometimes prescribed for children with bad epilepsy, when drugs have failed. It is by and large unpalatable and difficult to comply with, but it does help in a few cases.

Monitoring treatment

You and your doctor together need to check how your treatment is affecting you. You should give the doctor as much information about yourself as you can. The checklist on page 72 will help you.

People with epilepsy may have regular blood tests to monitor their treatment. For some drugs, phenytoin in particular, there is a range of blood concentrations below which the person might not be receiving the maximum benefit in suppressing seizures, and above which there are likely to be side effects. Although blood tests are unnecessary for most people, they are useful and may be essential for the following:

- people who still have seizures, whose doctors need to decide whether the dose of the drug they are taking can be increased or whether other drugs should be used

- people developing side effects, particularly if they are taking more than one drug

- special situations, such as pregnancy, liver or kidney failure, or

Monitoring your treatment with a doctor

1. Keep a diary of when seizures occur; their frequency and pattern of occurrence will influence treatment. Seizure diaries are available from hospitals, but any diary can be used.

2. Keep a record of different types of attack, and differentiate between them. Minor attacks that do not interfere with your lifestyle need less aggressive treatment than major attacks that do.

3. How do you feel about your medication? Are there any symptoms that you think might be caused by the drugs? Watch out for drowsiness, poor concentration or memory, and unsteadiness.

4. Have you had any new symptoms or illnesses since your last visit to the doctor?

5. If seizures have occurred unexpectedly, are there any special circumstances that might be responsible, such as missing your medication, a late night, alcohol?

6. Have you seen any other doctors (perhaps in a hospital casualty department) since your last visit to your regular doctor, and have any changes been made to your treatment?

7. Are there any questions about epilepsy that you want your doctor to answer? If so, make a list so you don't forget.

8. Even if you have been very well, ask your doctor to review your treatment every year. Don't simply continue to pick up repeat prescriptions.

for people who are mentally retarded, when drug intoxication may be difficult to detect

● to check whether a person is taking medication regularly and reliably.

Your doctor

People with epilepsy will come into contact with different kinds of doctors during the investigation into their illness. For your continuing treatment you must make sure that only one doctor supervises your checks and medication, and who this is must be clearly understood by everyone concerned. In the UK, for most people who have relatively mild epilepsy, the family doctor is the best person. People with more difficult problems might be put under the supervision of a specialist: a paediatrician for children, or a neurologist (a specialist in diseases that affect the nervous system) for older people. In the United States it is usual for the majority to be supervised by their own paediatrician or neurologist.

Specialist advice from a psychiatrist is helpful for people whose mental problems complicate their epilepsy.

Your relationship with your doctor is important You should feel confident that you can contact him or her when you need to discuss your condition and any worries you may have. You can also ask to be referred to a specialist, and you should discuss with your doctor who would be the best person.

Special centres

There are a number of special centres that offer rehabilitation in a carefully controlled environment for people with severe epilepsy (see page 119).

The activities are all those that are aimed at making people more independent. A major part of the work is getting people away from perhaps overprotective family environments. They teach people to make decisions for themselves, get on with new people, form relationships. Basic skills are taught that may be helpful in finding employment. They can also be useful in amending treatments and sorting out diagnoses, and very often they have an important role to play in helping people who have both epilepsy and psychiatric disturbances.

Epilepsy and other medical treatments

You must always inform doctors and dentists about your epilepsy when seeing them for other conditions. Your dentist, for example, will need to know if you are taking phenytoin, which can cause swelling of the gums. Your epilepsy or your medication might also influence whether you receive treatment in the dentist's surgery or in a local dental hospital.

It is safe for people with epilepsy to have surgical treatment for other conditions. Make sure that the surgeon, anaesthetist and medical staff know about your epilepsy and the drugs you take, and continue your regular medication during your stay in hospital.

Most immunizations are safe and you are encouraged to take them. The one possible exception is whooping cough vaccination. Sometimes status epilepticus (see page 77) and brain damage can occur after this vaccination, but similar problems are more common in children contracting whooping cough, and can happen for little apparent reason in others. It sometimes is said that children already known to have brain damage or epilepsy, or who have a close relative suffering from epilepsy, should not be immunized. If this is your child's situation, you need to consider immunization very carefully with your doctor.

6 THE OUTLOOK: CURE OR CONTROL?

One of the most important questions for people who have recently been diagnosed as having epilepsy, and for their families, is can the epilepsy be cured or controlled? The two are obviously different. Cure implies that the medication can be stopped eventually, with no likelihood of further attacks taking place. Control means that attacks may stop, but will probably return if the medication is withdrawn.

The overall outlook, or prognosis, for control and cure is good. Usually attacks can be prevented with drugs, and where this is not possible the number of attacks can in most cases be greatly reduced. Between 70 and 80 per cent of people who develop epilepsy will have a long period of remission of seizures, which lasts for many years, and about half of those whose seizures are completely controlled come off their drugs and remain free of attacks. Because virtually everyone who has epilepsy receives treatment with drugs, we cannot be sure whether the cure is a result of this treatment or due to the fact that some kinds of epilepsy occur only at certain ages and people can grow out of them.

Some people continue to have seizures throughout their lives, and need lifelong treatment with drugs. Why are these people different from the majority? The following factors seem to influence people's responses to treatment.

Type of seizures and epilepsy
This is probably the most important factor. Partial epilepsies are usually more difficult to control completely – approximately 50 per cent of people with this kind of epilepsy eventually stop having seizures – and complex partial epilepsy is the most difficult. Although drugs are very effective in preventing tonic–clonic attacks, they are much less effective against more minor partial seizures.

Children with some of the more severe generalized epilepsies, such as infantile spasms and Lennox–Gastaut Syndrome (see pages 35, 36), can also be difficult to treat.

The people with the best outlook have an idiopathic generalized epilepsy with a few tonic clonic seizures without an aura, or true petit mal. Ninety per cent of these people stop having attacks after they have been treated, and many are able to come off their drugs.

Age of onset
Epilepsy that begins in childhood almost always has a better prognosis than epilepsy that begins later: many childhood epilepsies disappear in adult life. The exception to this is epilepsy that begins in the first year or two of life, often after severe brain damage.

Symptomatic or idiopathic?
If the epilepsy is a symptom of brain disease, the chance of complete control is not good. People with brain damage usually have partial seizures, or symptomatic generalized epilepsies, and both these have a poor outlook.

These symptomatic epilepsies become more common in later life compared with others. This is probably the reason why age has become an important factor in the prognosis.

Duration and severity
The more frequent and longer the period over which seizures take place, the worse the outlook. For this reason some doctors believe that the sooner a person with epilepsy is treated, the better the outlook may be, and so they are eager to treat someone who has had only two seizures. Whether this early treatment really does influence the longterm outlook is controversial.

Taking all these factors into account, the best outlook is for children who have had only two or three generalized seizures (petit mal or grand mal) without an aura and who have no underlying brain disease or damage. The poorest outlook is for older people who have partial seizures that might be a symptom of some brain damage.

Compliance with treatment
One reason for failure to control fits is tablets being taken irregularly! It is important you remember to take your medication as prescribed (see also page 63).

76

Does epilepsy cause brain damage?

This is a common misconception. On the whole, people with epilepsy have IQs in the normal range, and many are above average. Some people who have suffered brain damage also have epilepsy and might be severely mentally retarded. Then the epilepsy, like the mental retardation, is a result, not a cause, of the brain damage. There are two extremely rare circumstances in which epilepsy can lead to brain damage:

1. Some of the severe childhood epilepsies – infantile spasms and Lennox–Gastaut Syndrome (see pages 35, 36) – can rarely occur in otherwise normal infants. These children may develop brain damage if the epilepsy is not controlled.

2. Brain damage can be caused by status epilepticus. The risk is greatest to children having prolonged febrile convulsions (see page 40). This is because the brain cells may become so overactive that the blood cannot transport enough oxygen to the brain to keep up with it, and so brain cells die.

Status epilepticus is a condition in which one tonic–clonic seizure succeeds another without the person regaining consciousness. When this continues for more than twenty minutes or half an hour it becomes potentially dangerous, threatening brain damage. The commonest reason why this happens to people who already have epilepsy is that they have stopped their drug treatment very suddenly.

7 EPILEPSY: FROM BABYHOOD TO OLD AGE

Having epilepsy has different implications depending on the type of epilepsy you have (see Chapter 3) and the age when the condition first appeared. In this chapter we discuss the worries many people have about how their epilepsy may affect them at different stages in their lives, both emotionally and physically.

Babies and young children

Having a baby diagnosed as having epilepsy will be upsetting for both parents. What you should never do is feel guilty about the condition having developed. No one is responsible for his or her genetic make-up. Brain damage caused at birth can be blamed on any number of reasons. It is futile and damaging for the whole family to spend time agonizing over these issues. The best thing for you and your baby is to establish as soon as you can a smooth running routine following your doctor's instructions on giving medication, and coping with fits with minimum upset and fuss.

How much protection should you give? I believe you should avoid restraint as much as possible. For a toddler or older child having sudden and unpredictable fits, a head protector like the one worn by the little boy in the photographs (page 80) may be necessary. These are lightweight and designed to be as uncumbersome possible.

Obviously there is a need for more supervision than with most children, and as your child grows and begins walking you will have to stop anything too dangerous such as climbing. Nevertheless, you must let your child explore his or her environment as much as possible as this is so important in learning and development.

Can you anticipate a seizure? This is difficult unless there are certain triggers that have been identified, or your baby has febrile convulsions (see page 40). Then you can avoid a fever by keeping the baby's temperature down with tepid sponging.

When do you explain the condition?
To your child   As soon as you think your child can begin to understand.   This is best not only because adjustment is easier if knowledge comes as naturally as possible, but also because your child will need to understand why regular medicine is necessary. Children should be encouraged to take their own medicine – under sensible supervision.

To friends and relatives   Again, as soon as possible.   This is particularly important for anyone who will be taking responsibility for your child at any time.

Schooling

At one time all children with epilepsy were considered seriously disabled and were educated in special schools. Now it is recognized that only a small number of children need to go to special schools, either because their seizures are so difficult to control or because they also suffer from other physical disabilities, or learning or behavioural problems. (The names and addresses of schools with specific facilities for children with epilepsy are listed on page 120.)

If it has been decided that your child can continue to attend an ordinary school, your first priority must be to tell the teachers about the epilepsy. You must be completely frank in discussing the condition with the teachers – they are no more likely to be well informed about epilepsy than anyone else who has no previous experience of it. All the teachers in the school must be aware that your child has epilepsy.

They need to know what might happen during a fit and what action to take (see page 28). If a seizure does happen at school, once the fit itself has subsided the teacher in charge should take your child to a quiet area to allow peaceful recovery. It is hardly ever necessary to send a child with epilepsy home. The school staff should be told about the medicine the doctor has prescribed, and whether they need to supervise a midday dose. If possible, of course, your child should take medication at home in the morning before going to school and in the evening after returning home.

You must emphasize that the school should avoid identifying

79

your child as being different from the other children. He or she must obey the school rules just the same as the rest of the children, and should take part in the fullest range of activities possible. Most children can take part in physical education, including sports and swimming, as long as the teacher in charge can provide enough supervision to cover any eventualities such as a possible fit. Your doctor will advise you about how much your child can and should do. It may be wise for children with epilepsy not to participate in climbing activities.

Ultimately, the care of your child and the activities undertaken during school hours will be the responsibility of the school staff. You, the parents, should be in constant contact so that you can discuss with the teachers any problems resulting from your child's epilepsy. Whenever any of you is uncertain as to the correct course of action you must seek advice from the doctor supervising your child. Schooling should be an enjoyable experience and one that will develop your child's talents to the full.

Adolescence

Anyone who has grown up with epilepsy from childhood should have adjusted to seizures and to taking medication. Other physical changes of adolescence can nevertheless affect your epilepsy and how you feel about it.

Will you have changing patterns of attacks? Seizures may change during adolescence. Petit mal seizures tend to become less frequent and children who have had these sometimes start to experience tonic–clonic seizures. Children with brain damage and symptomatic generalized epilepsy may start to have more classical complex partial seizures during the teenage years (see Chapter 3). Other influences that could bring on more attacks are the classic triggers: too little sleep and too much alcohol!

If you have just been diagnosed and are coping with the physical and emotional tensions everyone experiences in adolescence, having epilepsy may seem an impossible burden. You may be tempted to rebel against your condition and ignore medication and visits to your doctor. You won't be in a mood to welcome good advice. Nevertheless, this is not a time to withdraw

80

into your shell. It will be much easier to live with your epilepsy if you can talk about it openly:

- do find a doctor you feel you can communicate with

- do tell your friends about your condition and how to help you during a seizure

- don't restrict your life: follow your favourite pursuits – within reason. You will find there are surprisingly few that you can't enjoy.

Going to college

A lot of people with epilepsy go in for higher education. If you have won a place at a college or university you will need to make a few special preparations:

- Tell the college medical officer and your own tutor that you have epilepsy

- If possible, arrange to live in a hall of residence, at least for the first part of your course. This means you won't have to bother with cooking and domestic chores while you become used to studying. You will also have plenty of contact with other students, and know there are always people to help during a seizure.

- All examiners, internal and external, should be informed that you have epilepsy. They may need to make allowances for this when marking your papers, should a fit have occurred during an examination.

Does too much studying bring on a seizure? I don't believe this ever happens. But you must avoid falling into the trap of studying late at night. Lack of sleep certainly brings on fits.

Personal and sexual relationships

Some people with epilepsy do experience difficulty in getting along with schoolmates, friends and workmates – but so do many people who do not have epilepsy. The question that always arises is: whom should you tell that you have epilepsy? Often people are secretive about their epilepsy because they feel that it will alter people's attitudes towards them. Unfortunately, this can happen, but secrecy almost certainly perpetuates the myths and misunderstandings that

81

surround epilepsy, so that in the long term it is the wrong choice. The more people who realize that one of their friends, their teacher, a workmate, has epilepsy and is still a very able and active member of society, the less prejudice there is likely to be about it.

The ultimate test of anyone's success in forming personal relationships is likely to be marriage and family life. People with epilepsy can marry and bring up children with the same hope of success as anyone else. But the potential worries about contraception, pregnancy and inheritance are among the most frequent we hear about at our clinics.

Contraception

The oral contraceptive pill is still the most convenient and effective method of contraception for women with epilepsy. If you are used to taking medication, you are unlikely to forget the pill, and its success rate as a contraceptive is still high. However, certain anti-epileptic drugs – phenytoin, carbamazepine and phenobarbitone – affect the body's metabolism. This means that the active substances in the pill, the oestrogen hormones, are made inactive more quickly and efficiently than they would be otherwise. Very rarely this can result in unwanted pregnancies.

Most standard pills contain very low levels of oestrogen. If you experience bleeding between periods, which is a clear indication that not enough oestrogen is being taken into the body, you will need to take pills with a higher level of oestrogen to maintain the right level for effective contraception. Discuss this with your doctor or family planning clinic, who can make sure that you are taking the right strength of pill. Higher strength pills do not carry any additional risks for women with epilepsy. There is no evidence that taking the pill makes seizures better or worse.

There is increasing resistance to the pill because of possible, though as yet unproven, risks of heart disease or cancer. If you feel unhappy about taking the pill you can use one of the other means of contraception that are satisfactory for people with epilepsy. Your doctor or family planning clinic can advise you on what is best for you as an individual.

Pregnancy

What is the risk of having a child with epilepsy? Overall, between 1 in 100 and 1 in 200 of the population has epilepsy. If one parent has epilepsy, the risk for a child is about 1 in 40. If both parents have epilepsy, the risk is greater, about 1 in 10 to 1 in 5. These risks would seem to be quite acceptable, except in the very rare situation where epilepsy is just one of a number of disabilities that might be inherited. In these circumstances people need to seek specialist advice.

The risk for the population as a whole of a child having any physical abnormality is approximately 2 to 3 per cent. The risk to the child of a woman who is taking antiepileptic drugs is two to three times as great. Some of this increased risk can be attributed to drugs taken throughout the pregnancy. The drugs that have been identified as risky are the older ones, phenytoin, phenobarbitone, and possibly sodium valproate. Phenytoin and phenobarbitone have been associated with hare lip and cleft palate abnormalities, and with malformations of the heart. Fortunately, when these do occur, they often can be put right by an operation.

There has been some suggestion that sodium valproate can be associated with children being born with spina bifida. The risks of this seem to be low, but women who become pregnant while taking valproate need to be checked. Early in the pregnancy ultrasound tests, blood tests, and possibly amniocentesis (sampling the fluid around the baby) should be done so that parents can be reassured that the baby is developing satisfactorily.

Pregnancy should not present any special problems, although it is impossible to predict what will happen to each person. Some women do have seizures more frequently during pregnancy, but an equal number have them less frequently. The majority of women with epilepsy experience no major change.

Medication Before you get pregnant, you should discuss with your doctor whether the medication you are taking is the best and safest for a pregnancy, or whether you should stop taking drugs during these months. If you have not had any seizures for two or more years, you and your doctor should consider trying to attain a pregnancy that is entirely free from the effects of drugs. If, though, you are still prone to attacks, the usual advice is to continue treatment throughout your pregnancy. The risks to a pregnancy seem to be greater from having uncontrolled epilepsy without drugs than relatively well controlled epilepsy with drugs. It may be that some simple changes in your medication will reduce possible risks to your baby.

It is important that you have your pregnancy carefully monitored by both an obstetrician and the doctor who usually looks after your epilepsy. Sometimes problems can occur in the last three months of pregnancy, when concentrations of drugs in the blood can fall. If blood tests show this to be happening, it may be wise to increase the dose at this stage and to go back to the usual dose after your baby has been delivered.

Breast feeding while you are taking drugs is quite safe for almost all mothers, as only very small quantities of the drug will pass to your baby in the milk. The problem that can arise with breast feeding is disturbance of your sleep. If being short of sleep makes your fits more likely, perhaps the father, using a bottle, can help with some of the night-time feeding.

Looking after babies and small children

This can create some problems, but none of them is insurmountable as can be seen from Sue Usiskin's story in Chapter 10. If you are prone to quite frequent fits, you may need more help, perhaps from your husband and other members of the family, than would otherwise be the case. Take simple precautions:

- Change your baby on a mat on the floor rather than on a table. Make sure that fires, electrical appliances and other potential dangers are adequately guarded

- Consider using a playpen; this may help reduce the risk to your toddler during your seizures.

Family life

Naturally everyone in the family is going to be affected by one of you having epilepsy.

Children

Bear in mind the advice throughout this book, that you should lead as normal a life as possible, and this means that the person with epilepsy should not expect special treatment and overprotection from relatives. Children with epilepsy should be treated in the same way as any brother or sister. Their independence should be encouraged as far as is reasonable, and they must follow the normal rules,

84

particularly if there are other children in the family. Make as few allowances for epilepsy as possible, and don't allow it to be used as a means of manipulation; that will only cause greater longterm tensions within the family and problems of getting along with others for the person concerned.

Middle age
You may be relieved to know that the physical and emotional changes experienced during middle age – notably the menopause – should not make any difference to your epilepsy: that it will not cause you additional concern.

Elderly people
One disease of later years that may produce epilepsy, however, is stroke. Epilepsy can develop as a complication. We describe this more fully in Chapter 4.

An elderly relative with epilepsy can be a special worry, particularly as the condition can arise in people who are handicapped by strokes or premature aging such as senile dementia. With an elderly person who has these complicated disabilities, a degree of patience and understanding is essential.

Drug treatment is nearly always successful. However, the elderly are particularly sensitive to the side effects of antiepileptic drugs, which can cause unsteadiness, drowsiness and confusion. Talk to your doctor if this seems to have reached an unacceptable level. An adjustment in your relative's medication should be possible.

Is special nursing necessary? Epilepsy is rarely a major problem in old age. If a relative does become too ill or difficult to look after at home, this will probably be due to a combination of problems and your decision as to the best care will have to be taken after discussion with your doctor and the rest of the family.

8 LIVING WITH EPILEPSY

Having epilepsy is going to affect your everyday life but it shouldn't make such an enormous difference as you may at first think. Some commonsense precautions and restrictions may be needed but there is no need to deprive yourself unnecessarily of doing things. Obviously, everyone who has epilepsy is different and what may be risky for one person can be perfectly acceptable for another. In this chapter we give advice that we hope will be useful in helping you adapt to a lifestyle that is best for you as an individual. As a starting point, the table on page 88 lists guidelines that apply to everyone.

Work

A wide variety of jobs is open to people with epilepsy. Whether you are suited to a particular job depends both on your own talents and on the nature of your epilepsy. Indeed, your talents, qualifications and experience should be fully considered in relation to the job on offer before the effect of your epilepsy.

People with very infrequent seizures, or seizures that occur only at particular times of the day – such as during sleep or first thing in the morning – will find there are few jobs for which they cannot be considered. People with more severe epilepsy and frequent, unpredictable seizures probably have a more limited scope.

How do you find a job? The first step is to look at the same sources as everyone else – Job Centres, newspaper advertisements and employment agencies; for school and college leavers the careers advisory service.

There are also special sources of advice: for school leavers, the specialist careers officer; at a Job Centre people with epilepsy can request the help of the Disablement Resettlement Officer (DRO), who has special responsibility for people with a variety of disabilities. The DRO may be able to direct you to a specialized training scheme that will provide useful experience and training.

Practical guidelines for living with epilepsy

Do

- Ask for information and advice about your epilepsy and its treatment.

- Make the most of your talents.

- Consider carefully the risks to yourself and other people of undertaking specific activities. If in doubt, ask advice, but try to err on the side of living a full and active life.

- Take your medication regularly and as directed.

- Avoid specific circumstances that might make your fits more likely.

- Try to talk to people about your epilepsy and correct their misconceptions.

- Consider joining one of the epilepsy associations. They might be able to offer you help, and you might be able to help others.

- Consider helping with research into epilepsy either by taking part in clinical trials or by helping to raise money.

Don't

- Remain in ignorance.

- Use epilepsy as an excuse for not realizing your potential.

- Miss doses or take extra doses when you 'don't feel well'.

- Drink heavily or have too many late nights in a row.

- Keep teachers or employers in ignorance of your epilepsy.

Finally, the Employment Medical Advisory Service provides advice to people looking for work as well as to employers about jobs that may be suitable.

A big difficulty is knowing how much information to give to a prospective employer, and when. It is certainly necessary to say that you have or have had epilepsy, unless it was a very long time ago. Not doing so could lead to dismissal without any protection under the Employment Acts. Ideally, you should not have to declare you have epilepsy on an initial application form. The Civil Service is an ideal employer in this respect: it does not ask for medical information on the first application form, but only after the job has been offered. Your medical suitability is then decided by a doctor who is a specialist in occupational health. Unfortunately, not all employers are as satisfactory. Too often the declaration of epilepsy can lead to an application being rejected by someone who has little or no understanding of the condition. Before filling in an application form it might be worth trying to find out who will be making decisions about any medical aspects. Sometimes it may be reasonable to leave blank those parts of a first application form that require medical information. However, if you do this you must declare your epilepsy if you are offered employment.

Which jobs are unsuitable?

1. If you have had even a single epileptic seizure after the age of five, you will not be allowed to drive heavy goods or public service vehicles, taxis, trains or aircraft.

2. You should be careful about trying for jobs where you need to drive at all, as further seizures can lead to your losing your licence (see page 93).

3. Avoid jobs that involve working at heights.

4. If you have frequent seizures, you should avoid factory work and working with heavy machinery, although this sort of work should be possible if you have a less severe form of epilepsy. Any machinery must be adequately guarded, regardless of whether workers have epilepsy.

5. You will find it difficult to gain admission to schools of nursing and medicine. Individual schools follow different rules, and each case is considered on its merits, but people with epilepsy will not be able to practise surgery or anaesthesia.

6. A history of epilepsy will prevent admission to the armed services and police.

7. People in the armed services who develop epilepsy will usually be downgraded medically, which reduces their prospects of promotion.

8. You can teach most subjects if you have epilepsy, but there may be restrictions placed on teaching physical education, and swimming.

Although the Disabled Persons (Employment) Act of 1944 provides that employers with twenty or more employees have a duty to employ disabled people to fill at least 3 per cent of their workforce, it has never been enforced legally, so no one has to employ a person with epilepsy. You have to show yourself to have the appropriate talents and qualifications, and be willing to sell yourself in an interview. You may have to work harder to get the job you want than people without your condition. You are not alone. Other groups of people with different disadvantages have to overcome them too. The final achievement is greater for the effort put in. Resist the temptation to blame epilepsy for any failures. That is inclined to make you defeatist.

Leisure

You should use your common sense in deciding which leisure activities you can take up and, of course, take the same precautions as anyone else. Remember that an activity that might be relatively risk-free for one person may be unacceptable for someone with more severe epilepsy.

On the whole, seizures are less likely to happen when people are taking part in active pursuits than when they are sedentary or sleepy and although you could be injured accidentally during a seizure, this does not happen often. None the less, this means that you would be wise not to indulge in some activities that could lead to injury – such as parachute jumping, windsurfing, mountain climbing and ski jumping – and to take special care pursuing others:

- **Swimming** You should always be accompanied by another person who knows you have epilepsy, and is a strong swimmer who could come to your aid if you were to have an attack in the water. You can enjoy other water pursuits in the same way, with the exception of scuba diving, which is not advised.

- **Cycling** You can go cycling in similar circumstances. If you have fairly frequent seizures, avoid cycling on busy roads, and in any case always wear a special cycling helmet.

89

- **Riding** Riding horses is an acceptable activity even for people who have physical handicaps as well as epilepsy. Again, you should always ride in company. The organisation Riding for the Disabled provides facilities and there are local groups to supervise these activities.

- **Climbing** is generally to be avoided, but climbing trees is a highly pleasurable pursuit for many children and is difficult to prevent. You must make the dangers clear to your child and try to restrict climbing to safe sites – without being too much of a spoilsport.

- **Ball games,** such as football, rugby, cricket, rounders and netball, should be all right for most people who have epilepsy but no other physical disability.

People often mistakenly imagine there are risks attached to a number of activities. Most worries are over the flashing lights of discotheques, television screens, computers and VDUs. Remember that very few people with epilepsy have seizures provoked by these kinds of visual stimuli. If you are at all worried about this, talk to your doctor, who will be able to tell you whether your EEG records show any evidence of this sensitivity.

Support groups – are they helpful?
Before visiting a support group, you should be aware that they often have a lot of very severely epileptic people so they can be unrepresentative of the population with epilepsy. This may be rather frightening for someone who has recently developed epilepsy. You may meet some people there who are perhaps retarded or brain damaged or who have personality disorders. However, these groups are certainly helpful in providing someone with social contact who otherwise would become quite isolated.

More able people with epilepsy attending support groups can be a positive help and benefit to those with severe epilepsy. If your condition is relatively mild, this is one way you can do a lot of good to fellow sufferers.

Alcohol

Alcohol plays a role in many social activities, and you need to treat it with particular respect for two reasons:

1. The drugs that are used to treat epilepsy do not mix well with alcohol. They can make the effects of alcohol more marked.

2. Alcohol can make seizures more likely. You may well have a seizure a day or two after stopping a bout of heavy drinking.

While it is not necessary to be teetotal, you should have no more than one or two alcoholic drinks during the course of an evening. Sometimes the labels on bottles of drugs used to treat epilepsy state that the medication should not be taken with alcohol. As a result people sometimes make the mistake of not taking their drugs because they know they are going to have a drink. That is, of course, the worst of all possible situations; you must take your medication regularly.

Travel

International travel is increasingly common, and there is no reason why you should not enjoy trips and holidays abroad if you take a few sensible precautions. Make sure that:

- You have enough medication to last you through your stay abroad
- You have adequate medical insurance before you travel
- Medical facilities are available and you can afford them
- You can reclaim any medical expenses incurred in EEC countries by completing EEC form E111 before you travel.

Flying itself will not cause fits, but international travel often upsets regular sleeping times. If you are sensitive to sleep deprivation, try to plan flights that will lead to the least possible disturbance.

Driving

This is part of everyday life for many people, but the laws that govern the right of people with epilepsy to drive are extremely strict. Neither your own doctor nor the doctors in the medical department of the Driver and Vehicle Licensing Centre (DVLC) have any great discretion in the way that these rules are applied.

If you have epilepsy and you have had two or more seizures in the recent past, you will not be allowed to hold a driving licence until two years have gone by without any seizures. This means that even if you are having only relatively minor auras, you may not drive a car or motorcycle. The one exception to this rule is that people whose fits occur only during sleep may hold a driving licence if they have had fits only during sleep for a period of three years. You may not hold a heavy goods or public service vehicle licence if you have had a single epileptic seizure after the age of five years.

When you have been diagnosed as having epilepsy, your doctor will tell you about these regulations and explain how they apply to you. But it is your responsibility to inform the licensing authorities. The driving licence states that you must inform the DVLC at once if you have any disability that is or may become likely to affect your fitness as a driver. You should not drive in the period between informing the DVLC and receiving a reply.

After you have gone for two years without any attacks, you can apply for a driving licence. The DVLC will obtain information from your own doctor and almost certainly accept your application. Your licence will be reviewed at three-yearly intervals. If you have another seizure, you will lose the licence for two years.

It is vital that everyone observes these regulations, for the risks are very real. Unfortunately, some people still ignore the law. In a survey of 2000 road accidents that were due to the driver collapsing at the wheel, 50 per cent were caused by epilepsy. Of those caused by epilepsy, 70 per cent of the drivers had a previous history of the condition and had failed to inform the DVLC.

Insurance If you continue to drive after the diagnosis of epilepsy, not only are you doing so without a valid licence, but also without insurance cover. You must inform your insurance company of your epilepsy when you get your licence, or get it reinstated, or they may refuse to cover you for any liabilities.

Practical points for everyday like

Most people with epilepsy can live independently perfectly safely. There are a number of precautions you should always observe,

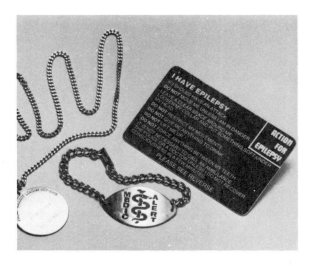

It is wise to wear a Medic - Alert or SOS bracelet or pendant, or carry an epilepsy information card.

whatever type of epilepsy you have, to guard against accidents during an unexpected seizure:

- Make sure your cooker and heaters, whether gas or electric (some people consider the latter less risky), are adequately guarded.

- When you are alone, shower rather than bathe if possible.

- Make sure that electrical leads from appliances and lamps are not left trailing about.

- Don't carry hot pans or kettles any distance; bring the plates to them.

- DIY should be safe for everyone except those with severe epilepsy, but do avoid climbing high ladders.

Living alone It is advisable to have a telephone at home. Although it won't be of much use during a seizure, it means that you can contact medical help should you need it afterwards.

If you have frequent fits, you might consider wearing a Medic-Alert or SOS bracelet or pendant, or carrying an epilepsy information card (see above). They can give important information to passers-by and hospital nurses and doctors if you have a fit in public when you are out alone.

9 RESEARCH

Our understanding of, and our ability to treat, epilepsy have improved dramatically in the last hundred years. At present the speed of advance is increasing and, although epilepsy is not a condition for which there is ever likely to be a sudden breakthrough that will produce a cure for everyone, we are optimistic that the outlook for people with epilepsy will improve considerably. Our increased understanding of how drugs are absorbed into the body and how they pass via the blood to the brain to have their action, how they are broken down and inactivated, has resulted in many improvements in the way existing drugs are used. The most obvious result for people with epilepsy has been the introduction of monitoring drug dosages by blood tests.

Until now all the drugs for treating epilepsy have been developed by screening programmes. This means that when a pharmaceutical company makes a new drug, it tests the effects on a wide variety of body functions. The drug is examined for its effects on some types of seizures on laboratory animals. Drugs that seem capable of preventing such seizures are then developed as antiepileptic drugs. We are now entering an exciting era. Our increased understanding of the basic mechanisms of seizures is leading to the development of drugs aimed at correcting the abnormalities that cause them.

Basic research

Many people are concerned about the use of animals in medical research. However, without animal experimentation we would not have gained our understanding of the cellular abnormalities underlying epilepsy, and it would not have been possible to develop any of the currently used antiepileptic drugs. Continuing progress in both these areas is heavily dependent on basic research being undertaken on laboratory animals.

Since the mid-1960s scientists have learnt a great deal more about the way in which neurotransmitters alter the behaviour of nerve cells (see page 12). At present the most exciting area of basic research concerns the neurotransmitter gamma aminobutyric acid (GABA), which has a widespread effect throughout the brain in decreasing the excitability of nerve cells. Our understanding of the way in which this neurotransmitter is synthesized within nerve cells, stored, released and inactivated has advanced enormously in the last ten years. We are beginning to recognize that many of the drugs that we use now, and which were discovered by chance, seem to have actions on GABA in the brain that might at least partly explain why they are effective in preventing seizures. We know that a variety of drugs that interfere with GABA in the brain can cause convulsions, and it seems that those that increase the activity of GABA can prevent seizures. Drugs are now being developed that increase the actions of GABA in the brain either by imitating it or by preventing its being broken down and so inactivated.

Scientists are also interested in a number of neurotransmitters that increase excitability in the brain, including glutamate and aspartate. Research is beginning into the possibility that excessive activity of these substances might have a role to play in producing epilepsy. By the mid-1990s newly developed drugs that interfere with the action of these substances will almost certainly be tested on people for their antiepileptic actions. While a lot of basic research is done in animals, all drugs must eventually be tested and found to be effective and safe for human beings. People with epilepsy can be directly involved in research by volunteering to take part in trials of new drugs.

There are at present many new drugs at various stages of evaluation. Although the majority will fall by the wayside for one reason or another, some will be found to be effective and safe, and will be approved for use in people with epilepsy. The first of these drugs has recently been licensed in the UK. Vigabatrin (Sabril) prevents the breakdown of GABA in the brain and so helps to prevent epileptic seizures. This is the first new drug to be licensed for epilepsy in sixteen years but it is likely to be followed by others in the near future.

Gabapentin is a drug which has a similar structure to GABA but it is uncertain whether its effect on reducing seizures is due to its effects on GABA.

Lamotrigine does not appear to work through GABA but it may reduce the action of excitatory neurotransmitters such as glutamate and aspartate. Both these drugs may have advantages in having

95

rather fewer side effects than some of the drugs currently used to treat epilepsy, and it is possible that they may be approved for treatment within the next two or three years.

New investigations

Over the last fifty years the most useful investigation for people with epilepsy has been the EEG. Advancing technology, particularly in electronics, has resulted in the development of telemetry and ambulatory monitoring (see pages 55-6), allowing more prolonged and useful recording. Undoubtedly, these advances will continue, and our ability to record the EEG over long periods with relatively little inconvenience to the people being tested will improve.

The major advances in investigations, however, are likely to come in ways of imaging the brain. Until now CT scanning (see pages 58) was the most important advance in this area, although it shows only the brain structure, and epilepsy is largely a disorder of the function of the brain that can occur without any structural abnormalities. The most exciting developments are new tests that examine the function of different regions of the brain. The first of these techniques is positron emission tomography (PET scanning).

For this test isotopes emitting positrons are injected into a blood vessel or inhaled. Low levels of radiation, which are no risk to the person being tested, are emitted by the isotope. These can be detected by special instruments. The data are then processed by computer to produce a picture that shows areas of high, or low, brain activity. The isotopes used are those of sugars or oxygen, which are taken up most by the most active areas of the brain. Trials with PET scanning seem to show that epileptic areas of the brain are less active between fits, and more active than the rest of the brain during fits. This test may prove to be helpful in identifying the areas of the brain that are a cause of seizures, and so improve the results of operations for the treatment of epilepsy.

A similar but much cheaper technique that is being used to investigate some people with epilepsy is SPECT scanning. This is rather similar to radio-active isotope scanning in which an isotope that emits single photons (a low level of radioactivity) is injected into a vein. This can be used to capture a picture of the blood flow of the brain. As parts of the brain that are damaged and give rise to seizures often have a poor blood supply between seizures and a high blood supply during and immediately after seizures, giving an appropriate isotope may help to pinpoint where fits begin. Because this technique needs only what is called a gamma camera, a machine which is available in many hospitals, research is being undertaken to see whether the use of this simple, cheap technique might simplify investigating people who are being considered for operations for their epilepsy.

The other new technique that is becoming available is magnetic resonance imaging (MRI). As with the other imaging investigations, this is done with little or no discomfort to the person concerned. Instead of x-rays or isotopes, a very large and extremely powerful magnet is used to take pictures of the brain, and produces images that are comparable to, and sometimes better than, those produced by CT scanning. This technology also lends itself to the investigation of brain function. It is likely that techniques using magnetic resonance can be developed to look at the activity of relatively small areas of the brain and examine their chemical make-up. Like PET scanning, this would improve our ability to define the abnormal parts of the brain that are causing the seizures.

Funds for research

It is important to understand how research into epilepsy is funded and what the problems are. The universities and government agencies are important sources of research funds in the United Kingdom. The major grant giving bodies are the Medical Research Council and the Department of Health. Other large charities also support research (The Wellcome Trust, The Nuffield Foundation, The Wolfson Trust). From these sources there is support for research into the basic mechanisms of epilepsy but unfortunately very little money is being spent on research into clinical aspects of epilepsy. A recent survey of the funding of research for neurological disorders in the United Kingdom suggested that if you had a rare condition such as muscular dystrophy anything up to £250 might be spent on research for every individual with that condition. For people with epilepsy the figure may be as little as 15p per person. It is unfortunately true that the funds available to the Medical Research Council and to universities have been significantly reduced in recent years, making funds for all kinds of medical research more difficult to obtain. It is also unfortunate that, unlike other conditions, the

Epilepsy Associations in the United Kingdom do not make up any of the gap that exists between the needs for research and the funding from the government. The drug industry is also a vital source of finance for research.

The drug industry is also a vital source of finance for research, and several large drug companies are actively involved in research into epilepsy and the development of new drugs for treating it. It would be very difficult to over-emphasize how important their contribution is. Although drug companies have at times been criticized for making excessive profits, the very stringent regulations that have to be met before a drug can come on to the market and be prescribed mean that drug development is an extremely expensive business. For every new antiepileptic drug that reaches the market in the next ten years, many hundreds will have been abandoned during the course of testing and development.

Perhaps most relevant to people with epilepsy and their families is the role played by charities in supporting research. Many large charities support research into brain function in general, and epilepsy in particular. You can contribute to the research funds of the national epilepsy association directly and through fund-raising events, and in this way contribute to advances in the treatment of epilepsy.

10 LIVING WITH EPILEPSY: A PERSONAL VIEW

by Sue Usiskin

The beginning

At fifteen the school art studio was the place I most loved to be. Looking back now, it seems ironic that it should have been here that my epilepsy started. As I sat at my easel absorbed by my painting, my eyes suddenly would not move from their fixed position. This strange feeling was swiftly followed by my head jerking to the right of its own accord. My right arm threw the paintbrush I was clutching into the air and I hear it land on the floorboards. I tried to call out but could not make any sound at all. I was falling backwards off my light metal chair. There was a loud crash, then blackness and silence.

We lived about thirty minutes from the school by car, so I was puzzled to see my father and mother leaning over me as I opened my eyes. My whole body ached, my head was throbbing and there were cuts on the backs of my hands. The studio was very quiet.

'Well, I'll be going now,' said an unfamiliar voice.

I turned my face in its direction to find the school doctor closing her bag. By her side stood the headmistress with a look of concern on her face. I was surprised to see her in the art studio; it was not a place she was usually to be found!

My parents took me home to bed where our family doctor came to see me. He checked my reflexes and my balance and we talked about what had happened to me. He suggested to my parents that I should see a neurologist and an appointment was made at a large hospital for the following week. I had no idea what to expect and felt more than a little apprehensive as we were ushered into the specialist's waiting room. I flicked through the pile of magazines with clammy, nervous hands. The minutes on the face of the wall clock ticked by slowly, punctuating the silence.

'The doctor will see you now, if you would like to follow me,' said a voice from the corridor.

My parents and I rose from our chairs and silently followed the receptionist into the doctor's consulting room. He stood up as we entered and extended his hand to my mother and father in turn. After the introductions, we sat down and he took notes on my general health and asked questions about my family history. He was fairly certain that what I had experienced in the art studio the previous week was an epileptic seizure, or fit. I would have to undergo a few tests at the hospital, after which he would see us again. He said that the treatment for my condition was 'not to have it'. I didn't understand what he meant by this and asked him to explain.

He sat back in his chair, folded his hands together and paused. Then, looking at me over the top of his spectacles, he said,

'It seems that you have had an epileptic seizure, but there is no reason why it should happen again, if, indeed, that was the case. It is possible to control it with medication, you see. Now, I want you to go and have an EEG and a head x-ray, and come back to see me in a week. By that time I shall have seen the test results and will be able to start you on a course of treatment. Is there anything else you would like to ask me before I take a look at you?'

' What is an EEG? I don't think I know.'

'It's short for electroencephalogram, which means a tracing from the impulses given out by the brain. Certain patterns tell us if there are problems and which areas of the brain they come from.'

I nodded and he rose from his chair and moved round to my side of the desk.

'Just stand up for me, will you?' he asked.

I stood and looked up at his face as he towered over me.

'Now, I want you to follow my finger with your left eye, keeping the other eye covered,' he said. 'Good. Now the other side.'

He continued his instructions and after about five minutes he told me to sit down again. Returning to his desk, he made a number of notes while I shifted in my chair in nervous anticipation. He put his pen down, sat back and looked across at my parents.

' Would you all like to come back here next week?'

They nodded.

'The tests can be done on Friday morning. I'll tell my secretary to arrange it for you. I should have the results early next week before you come back. I shall, of course, be writing to your doctor and to the school.'

He rose from his chair again and came round the desk towards us, holding out his hand. We thanked him for his help and said goodbye.

100

Some days later I went to have the tests. The first one was a simple x-ray of my head. It was followed by an EEG. For this the technician attached a number of electrodes to my scalp by means of long wires. By the time she was ready to record the pattern of my impulses, I must have looked rather like an astronaut! The whole process was entirely painless and quickly over. When we returned to see the doctor the following week he told my parents that he had seen all the test results and felt it would be a good idea to being my treatment immediately. He explained that it would take time for me to adjust to the antiepileptic drugs. In the event of any difficulty, I was to contact him.

Adjustments and side effects

It was, in fact, nine months before I had another seizure. I remember very little about this period of my life, mainly because the anticonvulsant regime that I had been prescribed made me feel vague and sleepy much of the time. The second seizure also happened at school. After I had recovered sufficiently to be moved down to the sick room, I lay wondering how often this was going to happen when I heard the familiar voice of my class teacher:

'I thought we had finished with all this.'

I was to learn that there are apparently no limits to what people say in this situation when they are ignorant about epilepsy.

Once again my parents were asked to come and collect me. I slept most of that day, waking only in order to take my anticonvulsant medication. My parents were anxious for me to contact my specialist, which I did. He suggested a slight increase in my medication and the addition of another drug. This, he felt, would give us better control of my seizures.

As the increased medication gradually took effect over the next few weeks I began to feel increasingly drowsy and unsteady. No amount of sleep made any difference. I expressed my concern to the doctor, but he said that I should continue the medication and my body would adjust in time. It didn't. I found myself living in the twilight world of sedation and I still had seizures from time to time. I have very little idea of how different my life would have been at that time had there been available then the plasma level tests that today so efficiently measure the concentrations of medication in the blood. One thing I do know for sure is that since the advent of these tests I have never again had to endure the misery of drug intoxication that I suffered then.

Until this time in my life I had a great many friends both at school and socially. My family recall that at this stage I became increasingly selective about the company I kept. My father saw it as my way of protecting myself. By getting out of social relationships first, I was in effect sparing myself the pain of possible rejection by others if they found it difficult to cope with my unpredictable condition. I think it was my first major fit in a public place that consolidated my fears of rejection.

It happened one evening while I was waiting for a bus with a group of friends. Afterwards I thought that being seen with me when I was having a fit might be a problem for my friends, as they might feel that it somehow reflected on them. It is true that for most people mid-adolescence is a time of acute self-consciousness, and for this reason alone the prospect of being seen with someone who suddenly collapses on the ground in a noisy, jerking heap was one pressure they could do without. Thus my social relationships became fewer and the consequent isolation aroused within me a sense of being different.

Life at home had been harmonious and the relationships between my parents, myself, my brother and two sisters were good. My father recalls that after the onset of my epilepsy my need for extra support had an unsettling effect on the other children, and they began to compete for attention in various ways. Just as my parents had been called to school in connection with my health, they were now being called to discuss emotional problems with my two younger sisters' teachers. At the time I was not aware of any connection between my own special needs and those being displayed by my sisters and brother.

My parents coped admirably with all the adjustments that these initial few years brought. They never tried to limit my activities because of what people might think if I had a fit, which would have been all too easy to do and would, I am sure, have saved them many anxious moments. I was fortunate that they were not overprotective, and I was not made to feel delicate or incapable. On the contrary, they realized that I needed to do more than accept my epilepsy if I was to develop into an integrated member of society. I was encouraged to make an extra effort to overcome my difficulties and not to allow them to become an excuse for doing less. In any longterm condition such as mine, it is vital to develop a positive attitude. If such an attitude isn't fostered in the beginning, it will become increasingly difficult to develop later. It is most important to have a coping strategy and to be able to share it with others, who will take their cue from you. This is not always easy to achieve but it improves with experience.

My school work began to be a problem. The drugs had severely reduced my ability to concentrate and I took a very long time to complete my homework every night. I would sit at my desk for hours, struggling to apply myself and finishing only a modest amount. Sometimes the effect of my drugs was so strong that I stared blankly out of the bedroom window in a dream. I would stir only at the sound of my mother's voice calling me to come down for supper. Despite these difficulties I managed to obtain seven O-level passes with reasonable grades. I did well in art, which had always been my best subject and the one I wished to pursue.

College days

My mother was a sculptor specializing in the human form, and she did quite a lot of portrait work. I had always spent a lot of time sitting in our garage where she worked, observing everything she did with interest, and learning a great deal. Growing up in this creative environment, it seemed natural that I should now apply to art college. I was delighted to hear that I had been accepted. My boyfriend was studying at the same art college, and we both belonged to an amateur drama group in our spare time. I had heard that in some cases spotlights act as a trigger in epilepsy and I think it was then that I had to make my first conscious decision about how my condition should affect my life in general. I used practical danger as my yardstick. If an activity put me in real physical danger, I would not risk it. For example, I loved riding horses, but I thought the chance of having an epileptic attack while doing so was not worth the risk. However, I did not believe that spotlights constituted a comparable danger and therefore did not avoid activities, such as the drama group, where they were present.

The last eighteen months had been important to me socially. I had begun to evaluate my health and realized that generally I remained quite healthy. This was a boost to my hitherto sagging self-confidence. It is true that 'nothing succeeds like success', and although I was still having fits, I was beginning to live with my epilepsy. I had been happy to discover that my condition did not appear to discourage boyfriends, as I had at first feared it might. On the contrary, they were pleased with a simple explanation and some practical tips. Perhaps it made them feel more protective towards me. I didn't really know; all that mattered to me was that they were not overtly worried by my revelation. My parents were obviously delighted by my refound gregarious personality and suggested that I give a party for my friends. I had been to many parties over the past months and this would be an opportunity to return some of the invitations. I was grateful for their suggestion and enjoyed the occasion with real enthusiasm.

While I was at college I became aware for the first time of just how other people saw epilepsy. I was called upon to help when a fellow student had a seizure in the college canteen one afternoon.

'So this is what they're so frightened about,' I thought, looking down at her rigidly convulsing body, which emitted strange grunting noises.

I had never realized how undignified having a fit could be and I found it hard to identify with what I witnessed. But I was sure it was this, combined with epilepsy's unpredictable nature, that other people found it difficult to cope with. After all, a seizure can happen any time, anywhere, which gives it a high nuisance value for you as well as for the onlooker. Never knowing when your next seizure will strike makes it very difficult to plan ahead. But no matter how hard you try to live from day to day, a certain amount of planning is necessary and desirable after all, it's just simpler that way. If you do have to drop out of something, you have to accept the fact and try to replan the activity for another time. It is highly unlikely that you will have to cancel the same thing twice.

Living on my own

I enjoyed my years at art college very much indeed. After one year on the foundation course, I applied to study jewellery design at another college, where a degree course was offered. To my delight, I was accepted and began to plan for the changes. It was to be the first of many changes in my life. I had been thinking about moving out of my family home, as I needed to be able to work uninterrupted and without disturbing anyone else. The only time I found I could do this was quite late in the evening when no one else was about. I would still be working in the small hours of the morning, completely absorbed by whatever I was doing. My bedroom was very small and I needed more space to spread out while working on a variety of design projects. I began to look for a place that would provide me with the extra space and my first opportunity to live on my own.

After some strenuous searching I went with my father to look at a small terraced cottage. It seemed to be ideal, providing a room where I could work downstairs and a bed-sitting room upstairs. My parents agreed to the proposed move and helped me to organize it. The encouragement they gave me at this time was remarkable considering how concerned they must have been about my living alone. However they felt, they supported my move with enthusiasm. I was extremely lucky, for their positive attitude enabled me to function at nineteen as an independent young adult, with sufficient confidence not to hide behind my health problem. I did not fully appreciate just how important this was until I met one of my neighbours.

One afternoon not long after I moved in I came home with some shopping. While searching for my keys, an unfamiliar voice greeted me.

'You must be the new neighbour.'

I turned around to find a pleasant-faced woman, who seemed quite out of breath.

'That hill, I'm sure it'll be the death of me,' she continued as she unbuttoned her raincoat, sighing deeply. She introduced herself, saying that she lived on my right with her husband and two daughters, then asked me to excuse her, as her elder daughter was at home not feeling well.

We met again within a few weeks and I inquired how her daughter was feeling. It was then that I learned why the girl was again not at work.

'She's had one of her turns again,' explained her mother. 'It's such a shame. She's had rather a lot lately.'

It soon became clear to me that the girl had epilepsy. Her mother was embarrassed about it, so she referred to it as 'turns', a euphemism I have often heard. Many people find they cannot get the word epilepsy past their lips. Although we have come a long way since the time when 'epileptics' were thought to be possessed by the devil and burned at the stake as witches, prejudice lingers on. Even the idea that epilepsy is a form of insanity still exists. When you begin to see why many people are so guarded about the condition, you can understand their plight.

Eventually, I met my neighbour's daughter. She found it difficult to relate to people and was extremely shy and withdrawn. It was clear that she had a profound sense of being different, but it was quite different from mine – there emanated from her an air of shame.

105

As I got to know the family better I saw that there was a definite link between her parents' inability to accept her condition and the way she coped with it. Because of their overprotection she had missed the opportunity to develop a positive attitude to her life and to emerge as a confident adult.

The years I spent at college while living on my own were very happy ones. I always felt self-contained in my home. I was often asked if I missed company and I would reply that as I worked with other people all day, I rather enjoyed being alone at night. I saw my friends and family when I wanted to and it seemed a perfect arrangement. I broadened my course at college to include fashion design and I worked hard, enjoying the greater variety in this department. I was still having problems with the side effects of my antiepileptic drugs, which slowed me down and affected my concentration. There were times when I felt thoroughly depressed, for although I was grateful for the measure of control over my seizures that the drugs afforded, it seemed to me a high price to pay in terms of dulled energy. My consultant did not appear to be concerned about this and even suggested I take a mild tranquillizer in addition to my other drugs to stop me worrying about the side effects! He assured me that this other drug he was prescribing also had antiepileptic properties and therefore might give a better degree of control over my seizures. I felt cornered. My instincts told me that the present 'cocktail' was sufficient, not to say excessive, but it had never given me the complete control I had hoped for. After much deliberation I agreed to try, but only because at the time I felt I was in no position to refuse. I wanted to be able to control my epilepsy.

In my last year at college I began to see a lot more of my boyfriend, Andrew. I had completed a collection of designs that I hoped to market, and he encouraged me to start work as a freelance fashion designer. My plan was eventually to set up a small fashion accessory business that I could run from my studio at home. It seemed to be a practical way of coping with my unpredictable health problem, as it meant I did not have to travel. I had been put off using the underground by one frightening experience. While going down a steep, crowded escalator at an underground station I felt a seizure start. It was the rush hour and I was packed in the crowd like the proverbial sardine in a tin. I found myself unable to move, locked firmly between the people standing in front of and behind me. In this way I was prevented from falling down the length of the

106

escalator. I had always hated crowds, but I realized then that they had their uses after all! Thereafter I reduced travelling to an absolute minimum. Escalators along with riding and climbing were 'not worth the risk'.

Marriage, pregnancy and medication

Whenever my epilepsy gave particular cause for concern I would tell my consultant, which he had always been eager for me to do. The problem was that his response would often be to increase my dose, sometimes prescribing additional drugs without monitoring their effect. It is no surprise that this way of dealing with my epilepsy proved to be disastrous. My general health suffered. It was not long before my condition had deteriorated markedly and I began to feel vacant and lethargic. Although it was difficult for me, I somehow managed to continue to run my small business from home, encouraged by Andrew.

Andrew had established a design business of his own, which he operated from a studio about two miles away. He designed shops, offices and showrooms, offering his clients contract supervision as well. This, with his enthusiasm for every design project, inspired confidence and his business grew steadily. We saw quite a lot of my family, who were very fond of him and therefore delighted to hear that we wanted to get married. We planned to have the wedding in March of the following year, when I would be twenty-two.

We both wanted to have children and thought it would be a good idea to talk to my doctor about the hereditary aspects of epilepsy. He said I had a 10 per cent chance of passing it on to our children. Andrew and I took the view that such a relatively small chance was worth taking. In any case, I continued to live with my epilepsy and saw no reason why, should the need arise, we could not help a child to do the same.

When I became pregnant, Andrew suggested that it would be best for me to attend the obstetric clinic at the same hospital where I was seen for my epilepsy. None the less, although I worried terribly about the effect of my frequent attacks on our unborn child, I was never warned of the effects my drugs could have on the baby. Happily, apart from being a month premature, our son, Oliver, was unaffected.

My fits were very frequent and I depended on Andrew for practical help when the baby arrived. He encouraged me to seek a second opinion. Looking back, I realize that if it had not been for his support, I might still be taking excessive doses of anti-epileptic drugs, unaware of any alternative. The first thing my new neurologist discovered was that I was grossly intoxicated by the antiepileptic regime I had been given over the years in ever-increasing amounts. In his opinion I was having more seizures because I was so run down by the treatment I had been receiving. Under his supervision my regime was simplified and reduced. I began to feel alive again, and my condition improved from having up to three seizures a day to about three a month.

Now I was able to look after Oliver. I was extremely disappointed that I could not breast feed him. I was told that the drugs I was taking would have affected my milk. This was in fact the wrong advice, and yet it turned out to be very convenient. It meant that Andrew could share the feeding, and if I was not well someone else could take over for a while. My approach was always practical. I never bathed Oliver when I was alone with him. This was a safety precaution that I always applied to myself as well, just in case of an attack, and one I adhere to still. I also doubled up on changing equipment to avoid having to carry the baby repeatedly up and down the stairs and I changed him while he lay on a mat on the floor rather than on a bed from which he might fall if I had an attack. Apart from these precautions, I set about caring for Oliver in just the same way as any other young mother.

Of course, we also took safety measures in the kitchen to minimize any risks. Though to date I have not had an accident while cooking, I always use casserole style saucepans, without long handles, because if I were to have an attack near the cooker I would be less likely to knock them over. Similarly, I have never used an eye-level grill, as during an attack it would be easy to pull the grill pan out too far and spill its contents over myself and others. My personal rule is never to cook on gas because of all the dangers that naked flames could bring.

I was delighted with the reduction in my seizures. The connection between the level of my medication and my condition was undeniable. The new consultant explained to us that it is possible to poison a person by exceeding a correct level of drugs in his or her blood. Toxins accumulate in this way and lead to other problems, such as the ones I had experienced. I was very grateful for his help.

It was not long before Oliver could pull himself up in his cot and our thoughts turned to moving from the tiny cottage. We still

108

wanted to retain the facility of a studio at home. As Andrew could run his business from anywhere, providing he had a telephone, a desk and a drawing board, he thought it would be a good idea if he were on hand in case I needed him. We eventually found a home with the space we needed. It was a great source of strength for me to know that Andrew was near, and there were many times when his help was really useful.

Helping the children to cope

As soon as Oliver was mobile we realized that he would need help if he were to grow up able to cope with my epilepsy. We found the best way was to give him a small task to perform while I was having a seizure. His contribution was to get a cloth to place under my face to absorb any saliva produced and at the same time prevent me from grazing myself as I lay there. In a very short time he was able to 'help Mummy' whenever the need arose. However, it wasn't so simple when we were out.

It seemed that however well Oliver was able to cope at home, as soon as we were out the odds were stacked against us. Most people are quite ignorant about epilepsy, and so the reaction to a fit is often unhelpful to say the least. When Oliver was about two years old, I had a seizure in a taxi. The driver took one look and yelled,

'Get out of my cab! Go on, get out. I'm not having any drunks in my cab.'

It was raining hard, but he opened the door and dragged me out, leaving me to have the fit in the wet street accompanied by a sobbing toddler. This kind of incident was bound to leave its mark on Oliver however well adjusted he seemed in other circumstances. We persevered, hoping that by giving him a framework within which to cope he would eventually grow in confidence.

During my first pregnancy I had still been taking large, debilitating doses of various antiepileptic drugs, so it was a relief when I became pregnant again to find that I suffered infinitely fewer seizures than before. None the less, the birth of our daughter marked the beginning of an intensely traumatic few years for both of us.

Anna was born with a congenital heart defect. When it was diagnosed, no indication could be given about her future, and as she looked terribly ill at this stage we were very anxious. I am sure that in addition to a mother's instinct to do everything to help her child I was able to bring another dimension to her life. I knew from my own experience how crucial the attitude of the parents can be in building up sufficient confidence in a child to make life as normal as possible and prevent him or her feeling isolated and inadequate. Andrew was marvellously supportive and his strength and positive attitude were key elements in Anna's progress. To the surprise and delight of the doctors, Anna had attained almost completely normal development for her age by the time she was three. From then on she grew from strength to strength.

When they were small, Oliver and Anna played games together like many young children. A favourite for them both was mummies and daddies. Anna was directed in her role as Mummy by her brother. Oliver's list of instructions was a source of great amusement to us.

'Anna, you're going shopping,' said Oliver.

Anna obligingly responded by carrying a shopping bag across the room.

'Now you go to buy some bread.'

Anna mimed buying bread and putting her purchase in the bag.

'Now you have a fit!'

At this command Anna's shopping expedition would stop. She dropped to the floor and proceeded to imitate my convulsions. There was a lot of shaking and groaning, accompanied by ample spitting. After this she would lie still until Oliver told her to get up and continue her shopping. They continued to play together in this way for many years and I am convinced that it helped them come to terms with my condition, which could otherwise have had a very inhibiting effect on them both.

When I think of some of the distressing situations we lived through as a direct result of my epilepsy, I cannot help feeling amazed at my family's resilience. One afternoon when Anna was about three years old, we were walking down the busy high street to meet Oliver from school when I began to have a seizure. In the confusion that must have followed poor Anna was left stranded in the street watching me being whisked away by an ambulance that had been sent for by a well-meaning passer-by. No one had noticed her in the crowd and she tearfully made her way to Oliver's school, knowing that there would be nobody to meet him. Fortunately, when she arrived someone took care of her, but this kind of experience had an unsettling effect on us all. Afterwards, she woke up twice nightly for six months just to make sure I was still there.

110

Out in public

I make a point of telling people I come into regular contact with about my epilepsy. I feel more at ease with people who know what to expect and they are grateful for the opportunity to ask me how best to help. Many people do not realize, for example, that it takes quite a while until I am able to speak again after an attack. If we have discussed this point beforehand, they they will be prepared for it. However, attacks do occur in public when there is no familiar face to put me at my ease and this can present problems.

I sometimes get a warning that an attack is imminent and then I try to get to a safe place at once. The first sign of a seizure in my case is that my eyes fix on something. I know that from the moment this happens I have just a few seconds until the attack is in full force. The next stage of the warning is a jerking of my eyes to one side, closely followed by my head and neck. I have trained myself to use this short time to get down flat in the least cluttered space – away from walls, furniture and sharp objects – in order to avoid injury.

On one occasion, I was passing a large post office when I felt unwell. I went inside and made my way past the long queue to where the staff were. I tried to attract their attention by tapping on the glass door marked Staff Only. I was feeling increasingly unwell when a young man came towards me from behind the counter.

'Can't you read?' he demanded curtly. 'Staff only!'

'Yes,' I said weakly, 'but I think I'm going to have a fit.' I got out my official epilepsy card, which I carry with me at all times, to show him. 'I just want to sit down quietly...' I began to explain.

'Then why don't you go back out on the street where you belong,' came the retort. With that he simply turned on his heels and walked away.

This kind of response is, of course, a result of ignorance and the fear that accompanies it. I dare say that to this young man I appeared a nuisance, nothing more, but at the time his manner was distressing to me. His couldn't-care-less attitude put him in the same category as those who push past elderly people trying to get on a bus. Fortunately, I have also encountered people who are kind and helpful.

One fine spring day I was walking towards our local shops when I felt the first signs of an attack. There was no one in sight as I lay down on the pavement, trying to cradle my head in my arms. I heard a vehicle braking sharply near by, followed by quick footsteps. The attack gained momentum and as it did I became aware of someone kneeling over me.

'It's okay, love,' he said. 'I'll wait with you.'

Some time elapsed and as the seizure neared its final phase, the young man assured me that I was all right and must not worry. I lay in a daze on the pavement until he suggested that I might be more comfortable if I sat in his van for a while. I looked around for my handbag, still feeling dazed as he helped me to my feet. It certainly was more comfortable sitting in the van. The young man now assured me that he was not in a hurry and would wait with me until I felt well enough to go home. He seemed genuinely concerned for my welfare and his kind, gentle manner put me at my ease.

When I felt a little better, he offered to drive me home. I am not in the habit of accepting lifts from strangers, but this young man's caring manner filled me with confidence. He drove the half mile to my home and helped me down from his van.

'Hope you feel better soon, then,' he called as he turned to go.

On various other occasions I have derived quite a bit of amusement from the things people say while I'm having an attack. Unless I lose consciousness, I can hear what is going on around me. I realize that to many people the fact that the children are so calm and practical while their mother is out of control is in itself difficult to grasp. For Oliver and Anna the most pressing task is to try to persuade them that it is not the first time I have had a seizure, that I will recover, and that there is no need to send for an ambulance. Quite how loath people are to believe what a child says in this sort of situation was clearly demonstrated in an episode a few years ago.

I was in the local butcher's shop when I had a seizure. Oliver was kneeling down in the sawdust trying to look after me when I heard a customer say,

'Does mother often do this?'

When his reply was affirmative, she became quite indignant.

'Really? Are you sure?' as if he were trying to lead her on! To this woman it was utterly unbelievable: not only was I shaking, groaning and foaming on the floor but, according to my son, I did it often.

There are times when I feel that my condition imposes a considerable burden on the children. It is easy to attribute more or less all the emotional difficulties that my growing children experience to my health. One has to be aware of certain things that can be linked firmly to living with epilepsy. Oliver went through a phase when if he and I were to go out alone together, he would become rather tense and constantly ask me how I felt. He was clearly worried by the responsibility on his young shoulders. When I noticed this, I tried to include other friends on outings so that he was not alone with me. This appeared to help by providing a diversion for him.

Both Oliver and Anna have gone through periods when they repeatedly ask me how I am. It is not surprising, as they know only too well the risky nature of my life. Even with the correct level of anticonvulsants, I still have an average of three attacks a month. I would be surprised if my children showed no concern and the fact that they do not feel they need to make a secret of it can only be good.

One of the most difficult things that the children have had to learn to deal with is other people's tendency to want to rush me off to hospital. Over the years they have learned to be persuasive and, with the help of my official epilepsy card to back them up, they usually manage to convince members of the public that an ambulance is not necessary.

When the children are at school and I am out on my own, anything can happen. I was walking along our local shopping street on a particularly wet and wintry afternoon when I felt the first signs of a seizure developing. As usual, I tried to get myself to a reasonably safe place at once. I leaned heavily against the glass door of the nearest shop, a building society. Beckoning for help, I crumpled slowly to the floor as I entered. The attack gained momentum. I felt very conspicuous as, apart from myself, the shop was empty. The staff stayed exactly where they were behind the counter. Not one of them came around to where I lay shaking and groaning on the floor.

As the seizure finally subsided, I lay wondering how I might get one of the staff to telephone my husband at his office around the corner. (Since both children were now at school Andrew had taken an office locally, which meant he was still available in an emergency.) After a while I began to pull myself across the floor towards the counter. I fumbled in my bag and managed to retrieve my card from it. I indicated Andrew's number on the card. He came to the shop in no time at all. I was certainly very pleased to see him! The manager, who was still behind the counter, explained that he thought I was the 'front', the diversion, for a robbery, and had he come to my aid there would have been a chance for an accomplice to get behind the counter. I sat on the floor in complete disbelief. Andrew explained that my condition was quite genuine. The manager told us that he couldn't take any risks, and he seemed adamant about it.

The following day on my way to meet Anna at school I stopped at the building society to give the manager an information sheet called *Facts about Fits.* This is something I try to do whenever possible in an attempt to overcome the ignorance one usually meets. I have to admit I felt a bit silly, knowing that company's policy on coming to one's aid, but as I pointed out to the manager, a seizure can happen any time, anywhere, and it would be helpful to him to know how to give practical aid.

There are times when it would be easy for me to lose faith in human nature, so it is encouraging for me to recall the following incident, which took place in a branch of Marks and Spencer. As I walked through the food store wheeling a trolley in front of me, I began to feel the first signs that an attack was imminent. I approached an elderly gentleman who was busy filling up the shelves and touched him lightly on the shoulder.

'Excuse me,' I said, 'but I am going to have a fit.'

'Don't you worry, love, I'll help you,' he assured me. As he spoke he gently helped me down to the floor. He tore off a section of the package he had in his hand, folded it up and wedged it between my side teeth.

'There, love, bite on that,' he said.

Many people seem convinced that they should give you the handle of a teaspoon to bite on; this happened to me once and thanks only to the skill of my dentist the resulting chips were soon repaired. It is very dangerous to introduce any hard object into the mouth during an attack. The best thing to do is place the corner of a towel or handkerchief (not tissues) between the molars on the side the person is lying on. That way the airway is kept free.

When the attack had subsided, the staff helped me into a wheelchair and I was taken to their recovery room, where I could lie down in peace while they made me ample cups of tea. They told me that their doctor was on his way just to check me over before I went home. When he arrived, I felt almost human again, thanks to their expert care and kindness. Following a brief examination and chat, the doctor agreed that I was well enough to go. As soon as I was ready, the staff helped me into a taxi. They had even taken the

114

trouble to pack up my groceries for me.

As soon as I got home I composed a letter to the head office of Marks and Spencer – most people are quick to complain, but slow to praise. I described the way their staff had coped and how much this had impressed me. If more companies could learn from their excellent example, then people like me would have a far easier time.

There is a section of the public who are convinced that they know just what to do. They very often have a fixed but mistaken idea of how to help, which they announce loudly to all and sundry. Even if I do not like the sound of their plan of action, it is a matter of luck whether I am able to do anything to stop them. On one occasion I was lying on the floor in the reception area of a hairdressing salon. My attack was gaining momentum when I heard a woman announce that she knew exactly what to do.

'You have to pull out her tongue and hang on to it while you slap her around the face.'

I was horrified. Although unable to speak, I knew I had to try to prevent this imminent assault. This is easier said than done in the midst of a seizure. As my assailant leaned over me, I summoned up all my strength and kicked her. At the same time I made as much noise as possible in the hope that she would take the hint. The attack began to subside and by the time I was able to look around, she had gone. I pulled myself up and sat on a chair. Someone offered me a cup of tea, which I accepted gratefully. Tea is always appreciated after a fit, mainly for its comfort value – there is nothing comforting about a glass of cold water, which I have been offered time and time again.

Injury

One of the worst aspects of living with epilepsy is that you injure yourself quite often. The injuries can be divided into those you can take steps to prevent and those you can't. In order to minimize the potential danger from the force of my convulsions, I keep myself fit and supple with lots of exercise. If you have any condition that makes extra demands on your body in a great many ways, you have to work towards meeting them. Apart from the obvious benefit to muscle tone, exercise also increases stamina – something I find I need plenty of! It helps to shorten the time needed to recover from an attack. However, no amount of exercise can prevent head injuries. These are most likely to happen in the street, a singularly

115

unsympathetic place for a seizure. Usually the damage is quite minor. The bruises and grazes look a lot worse than they really are, but it is still depressing to have a visible reminder of an unpleasant event.

Other cures

Over the years I have never closed my mind to the possibility of an unorthodox cure. I've tried vegetarianism, teetotalism, caffeine- and tannin-free drinks, but the only effects I observed were anti-social ones. After reasonable trial periods, each lasting about six months, I would resume my former habits.

One day I heard that good results had been achieved by a healer using prayer and meditation. The instructions seemed odd, to say the least. I had to buy six lemons and six chillies and place them under my bed in their brown paper bag. Each day I had to sit looking at a photograph of the healer with a candle burning in front of it and recite the Lord's Prayer with my feet in a bowl of water. Every four days my husband had to take the paper bag and its contents from beneath our bed and drive to a nearby river and it had to be one that eventually opened into the sea. Here, looking over his shoulder lest he be arrested for dumping, he was to commit the contents of the bag to a watery journey. After continuing this for some weeks, the plan was laid to rest.

Prejudice and education

I am sometimes intrigued by what other people see as the major pitfalls of living with epilepsy. One evening when we were at a small party, the host said to me,

'You must get awfully fed up with wearing trousers all the time, Sue.'

I was completely mystified. What on earth did he mean? He had not said 'the trousers', but just 'trousers'. The expression on my face must have indicated my confusion, as he added,

'Well, you can't wear a skirt because if you have a fit, people might see your knickers.'

I was amazed by his notion, and told him laughingly that it had never occurred to me. Honestly, that is the last thing I would worry about when having an attack. He seemed quite surprised at this.

'So you do wear skirts?'

'Of course,' I replied.'I wear anything I like.' It seemed very strange that anyone should have thought up a special uniform for me.

On another occasion an elderly man said that I must have been very grateful to Andrew for marrying me. I responded that I was very happy, but saw no reason to be grateful. He replied that he did not think many people would want to marry someone with epilepsy. I explained that we led a normal life – punctuated by my seizures but otherwise normal – and I saw no reason to feel grateful in the sense that he implied.

What can be done about all the prejudice that still exists today? The answer must lie primarily in education. Young people need to grow up more able to cope with the wide variety of health problems they might experience in their lifetimes. It is my experience that young people have a natural interest in health matters, and what better place to satisfy this than at school? A compulsory course that teaches them how to give first aid, with a thorough grounding in all aspects of health education, would be a step in the right direction. Video tapes and slides could be used, and could form the basis for discussions. This would go a long way towards removing ignorance and fear, and so promote greater understanding and tolerance.

I speak to groups of doctors, nurses and medical students on the wide variety of problems that living with epilepsy presents. I emphasize that while it is often a source of stress, it can be a means of uniting and strengthening family relationships. It can help one keep a balanced perspective on life and not take things for granted. A student asked me recently if I felt that epilepsy had given me anything positive. My answer to him was that I don't get upset when the washing machine breaks down. Things assume a different scale of importance, and I am thankful for that.

In a school essay titled 'Relatives and how to cope with them', Oliver wrote:

My Mum has a thing called epilepsy, in other words epileptic fits. Every month or so she has them. It is hard to see your own mother lying on the ground shaking and foaming at the mouth but I have found that, hard as it is, just think how lucky you are it is not you. I know I have lots of things to worry about but I have learnt how to cope with them, so I'm not that unlucky.

When I read this, I was encouraged to find that Oliver was able to see things in such a mature way at his young age.

When I read this, I was encouraged to find that Oliver was able to see things in such a mature way at his young age.

Today, much can be done to help people with epilepsy. About 70 per cent will eventually achieve complete control on their medication, while 30 per cent may have to live with active seizures. The latter group in particular may encounter problems that are not generally dealt with in hospital clinics. A doctor may not realize that an anxious patient may be unable to absorb much information. Repeated interviews are often necessary to deal with such issues as fear, anger, denial and confusion. Continuity of care is important in establishing good communication and a feeling of trust.

People often have misconceptions about their epilepsy which they find difficult to introduce into a conversation with their doctor or counsellor. These include the association of epilepsy with mental disorders, presumed inheritance and the effect of seizures. It is important to discuss these aspects openly so that patients do not add to the burden of their condition by keeping their facts hidden.

An experienced counsellor, familiar with the difficulties people with epilepsy may suffer with their careers, social lives, family relationships and self-esteem, can have much to offer. He or she can address problems and give facts and reassurance. With the use of coping strategies to help build confidence, a positive attitude may be encouraged, general anxiety levels lowered and quality of life for the person improved.

Epilepsy can be lived with. The problems it brings are often trying but with a positive attitude they can be overcome.

USEFUL ADDRESSES

UNITED KINGDOM

The British Epilepsy Associations

72A London St
Reading
Berks RG1 4SJ
Tel: 0734 587345

Anstey House
40 Hanover Square
Leeds
Yorks LS3 1BE
Tel: 0532 439393 — for
  membership, talks and
  enquiries.0345 089599
  — National Information
  Centre

The Old Post-Graduate Centre
Belfast City Hospital
Lisborne Rd
Belfast BT9 7AB
Tel: 0232 248414

48 Govan Rd
Glasgow GS1 1JR
Tel: 041 427 4911

13 Guthrie St
Edinburgh EH1 1JG
Tel: 031 226 5428

Mersey Region Epilepsy
Association
'J' Block
Walton Hospital
Rice Lane
Liverpool L9 1AE
Tel: 051 525 3069

Wales Epilepsy Association
Gwynedd Voluntary Services
  Council
Eldon Square
Dolgellau
Gwynedd
Tel: 0341 422575

BEA Information Service
(24 hours)

BEA Membership/ Services	0898 777264
Facts about Epilepsy	0898 777265
Initial Diagnosis	0898 777266
Epilepsy and the Elderly	0898 777267
Epilepsy and the Child	0898 777268
Epilepsy and Driving	0898 777269
First Aid	0898 777270
Medical Management	0898 777271
Epilepsy and Employment	0898 777272
Epilepsy, Sport and Leisure	0898 777273

119

Callers charged 38p per minute
peak rate and 25p per minute off
peak. Callers may leave their
names and addresses at the end
of each tape, and literature on
the relevant topic will be posted
from the National Information
Centre.

Irish Epilepsy Association
249 Crumlin Rd
Dublin W12
Tel: 0001 516500

Epilepsy Helpline
0345 089599 (cost of local call)
9am–4.30pm Mon–Thurs
9am–4pm Fridays

The National Society for Epilepsy
Chalfont Centre
Chalfont St Peter
Gerrards Cross
Bucks SL9 0RJ
Tel: 02407 3991

Residential Centres for People with Epilepsy

Chalfont Centre for Epilepsy
Chalfont St Peter
Bucks SL9 0RJ
Tel: 02407 3991

David Lewis Centre
Alderley Edge
Cheshire SK9 7UD
Tel: 056587 2613

Meath Home for Women and Girls with Epilepsy
Westbrook Road
Godalming
Surrey GU7 2QJ
Tel: 04868 5095

The Maghull Homes
The Bartlett Home
Liverpool Road South
Maghull
Merseyside L31 8BR
Tel: 051 526 4133

120

Quarrier's Homes
Bridge of Weir
Renfrewshire PA11 3SA
Tel: 0505 612224

St Elizabeth's School
Much Hadham
Herts SG10 6EW
Tel: 027984 3451

Assessment Centres for Epilepsy

Bootham Park Hospital
Bootham
York YO3 7BY
Tel: 0904 54664

Chalfont Centre for Epilepsy
Chalfont St Peter
Bucks SL9 0RJ
Tel: 02407 3991

David Lewis Centre*
Alderley Edge
Cheshire SK9 7UD
Tel: 056587 2613

Maudsley Hospital – Epilepsy Unit*
Denmark Hill
London SE5 8AZ
Tel: 071-703 6333

Park Hospital for Children
Old Road
Headington
Oxford OX3 7LQ
Tel: 0865 245651

Not designated as a special assessment centre but provides an assessment facility.

Schools for Children with Epilepsy

Lingfield Hospital School
St Piers Lane
Lingfield
Surrey   RH7 6PN

St Elizabeth's School
South End
Much Hadham
Herts   SG10 6EW

The David Lewis Centre
Warford
Alderly Edge
Cheshire   SK9 7UD

Special Bracelets or Pendants

S.O.S. Talisman
212 – 220 Regents Park Road
London   N3 3HP

Medic-Alert Foundation
11/13 Clifton Terrace
London   N4 3JP

AUSTRALIA

National Epilepsy Association of Australia
Mr. Robert Gourley
Executive Director
PO Box 554
Lilydale Vic 3140

Epilepsy Association of the Australian Capital Territory Inc.
Shout Office
Hughes Community Centre
Wisdom Street
Hughes   A.C.T. 2605

Epilepsy Association of New South Wales
468 Pennant Hills Road
Pennant Hills
N.S.W.   2120
P.O. Box 521
Pennant Hills   N.S.W. 2120

Epilepsy Association of Queensland
Room 438
Penney's Building
210 Queen Street
Brisbane   Qld 4000

Epilepsy Association of South Australia Inc.
471 Regency Road
Prospect   S.A. 5082
P.O. Box 596
Prospect East   S.A. 5082

Epilepsy Association of Tasmania Inc.
86 Hampden Road
Battery Point
Hobart   Tas 7000
P.O. Box 421
Sandy Bay   Tas 7005

Epilepsy Association of Victoria
818–822 Burke Road
Camberwell   Vic 3124

West Australian Epilepsy Association (Inc.)
14 Bagot Road
Subiaco   W.A.   6008

121

ACKNOWLEDGMENTS

I thank all my patients with epilepsy, without whose help this book would never have been written. I should also like to thank Mr Peter Rogan for his help and advice on schooling and epilepsy.

DC

I thank Dr Gerald Stern for his consistent encouragement over many years, and Dr Simon Shorvon for the opportunity to counsel his patients from whom I have learned so much.

SU

The publishers would like to thank the following for their help in the preparation of this book:
Medic–Alert Foundation, London and Solport Ltd, Worthing, Sussex for lending equipment for photographs. The photographs on pages 26–7, 67 and 94 were taken by Ray Moller, assisted by Sophie Butt.
   The diagrams are by Kevin Marks.

INDEX

Page numbers in *italic* refer to the illustrations

Other books in the Positive Health Guide Series

Positive Health Guides: 'A series that gives health education a good name.' *British Medical Journal*

STROKE
A practical guide towards recovery
Dr Richard Langton Hewer and Dr Derick T. Wade
ISBN 0 356 14454 2

DON'T PANIC
A guide to overcoming panic attacks
Sue Breton
ISBN 0 356 14451 8

DIABETIC DELIGHTS
Cakes, biscuits and desserts
Jane Suthering and Sue Lousley
ISBN 0 356 14455 0

THE DIABETICS' INTERNATIONAL DIET BOOK
Ann Watson and Sue Lousley
ISBN 0 356 14739 8

DIABETES: A BEYOND BASICS GUIDE
Dr Rowan Hillson
ISBN 0 356 14850 5

THE HEALTHY HEART DIET BOOK
Enjoy delicious low-fat, high-fibre recipes
Roberta Longstaff, SRD and Dr Jim Mann
ISBN 0 356 14488 7

BEAT HEART DISEASE!
A cardiologist explains how you can help your heart and enjoy a healthier life
Prof Risteard Mulcahy
ISBN 0 356 19670 4

HIGH BLOOD PRESSURE
What it means for you, and how to control it
Dr Eoin O'Brien and Prof Kevin O'Malley
ISBN 0 356 14489 5

THE DIABETICS' DIET BOOK
A new high-fibre eating programme
Dr Jim Mann and the Oxford Dietetic Group
ISBN 0 356 14475 5

THE DIABETICS' COOKBOOK
Delicious new recipes for entertaining and all the family
Roberta Longstaff, SRD and Dr Jim Mann
ISBN 0 356 14474 7

THE DIABETICS' GET FIT BOOK
The complete home workout
Jacki Winter
Introduction by Dr Barbara Boucher
ISBN 0 356 14477 1

DIABETES
A practical new guide to
healthy living
Dr Jim Anderson

THE HIGH-FIBRE
COOKBOOK
Recipes for Good Health
Pamela Westland
Introduction by Dr Denis Burkitt

DON'T FORGET FIBRE IN
YOUR DIET
To help avoid many of our
commonest diseases
Dr Denis Burkitt

THE SALT-FREE DIET BOOK
An appetizing way to help
reduce high blood pressure
Dr Graham MacGregor

KEEPING BABIES AND
CHILDREN HEALTHY
A parents' practical handbook to
common ailments
Dr Bernard Valman

CHILDREN'S PROBLEMS
A parents' guide to
understanding and tackling them
Dr Bryan Lask

THE HYPERACTIVE CHILD
A parents' guide
Dr Eric Taylor

CONTACT LENSES
A guide to successful wear
and care
Professor Hikaru Hamano and
Professor Montague Ruben